PAIN:
FORGIVE,
LOVE,
HEAL

RAJIV PARTI, M.D.

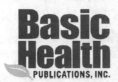

Basic
Health
PUBLICATIONS, INC.

The information contained in this book is based upon the research and personal and professional experiences of the author. It is not intended as a substitute for consulting with your physician or other healthcare provider. Any attempt to diagnose and treat an illness should be done under the direction of a healthcare professional.

The publisher does not advocate the use of any particular healthcare protocol but believes the information in this book should be available to the public. The publisher and author are not responsible for any adverse effects or consequences resulting from the use of the suggestions, preparations, or procedures discussed in this book. Should the reader have any questions concerning the appropriateness of any procedures or preparation mentioned, the author and the publisher strongly suggest consulting a professional healthcare advisor.

Basic Health Publications, Inc.

28812 Top of the World Drive
Laguna Beach, CA 92651
949-715-7327 · www.basichealthpub.com

Library of Congress Cataloging-in-Publication Data

Parti, Rajiv.
   Pain : forgive, love, heal / Rajiv Parti, M.D.
     pages cm
   Includes bibliographical references and index.
   ISBN 978-1-59120-355-1
  1. Pain—Psychological aspects. 2. Medication abuse—Patients—Rehabilitation.
3. Medicine, Ayurvedic. 4. Mind and body. I. Title.
   RB127.P3678 2014
   616'.0472--dc23
                                 2013039241

Editor: Susan E. Davis
Typesetting/Book design: Gary A. Rosenberg * www.thebookcouple.com
Cover design: Mike Stromberg

Printed in the United States of America

10 9 8 7 6 5 4 3 2 1

CONTENTS

To my parents
and to Arpana Parti,
my wife.

ACKNOWLEDGMENTS

Many people have helped in the creation of this book. I am deeply grateful to my teachers, my patients, my colleagues, and the physicians and medical staff who provided me with life-saving care.

I would also like to thank Bill Gladstone, my literary agent, and editors Mitch Sisskind and Susan E. Davis who helped prepare the book for publication.

PART ONE

PAIN AND ITS MEANINGS

Human beings are meant to be healthy. In body, mind, and spirit, we are designed for wellbeing. But this is not an end in itself. We are meant by nature to love and be loved, and good health is the environment in which this destiny can best be fulfilled.

But so many of us live in pain. Chronic or acute, physical or emotional, pain in one form or another is the cause of medical appointments involving millions of people every day. Yet in the majority of appointments involving chronic pain, no specific physical cause can be found. Why is this? How can this be? What can we do about it?

We can *forgive*. We can *love*. We can *heal*. But to do this with strength and understanding, we must first look closely at pain and the role it plays in our lives.

1

"I FEEL YOUR PAIN"

President Bill Clinton spoke those words at a public event in 1992. He was responding to a comment from a man who felt that the government was not sufficiently responsive to the AIDS crisis in the United States. Ever since then, *"I feel your pain"* has been one of Bill Clinton's signature quotes. But can one person really feel another person's pain? Can one person know what another person is feeling, whether it's pain, love, hunger, fear, or anything else? I'm not really sure. But the subject of this book is how to *end* your pain, not for me to feel it. And ending pain is an area in which I have experience as a board certified physician in anesthesiology and pain management—and also as a cancer patient who underwent surgery, chemotherapy, and eventual dependency on painkilling drugs.

I am a first-generation immigrant from India who just a few years ago was living the so-called American Dream in California. I had an expensive 10,000-square-foot home on a lake and an exclusive golf course. I was chief of anesthesia at a nearby hospital. I loved my work. Caring for patients undergoing heart surgery was my passion. The more challenging the case, the more satisfied I felt after doing a good job. My biggest satisfaction used to come when I made rounds in the morning and saw surgery patients having breakfast with a loved one. Sometimes I wondered if they had any idea how deeply at risk their life was for a time—for example, when we in the operating theater were having difficulty jump-starting their hearts after a long "pump run."

I had expensive cars, and got a new one every few years. Often I would kid with my friends, "I can't change my wife, but at least I can change my cars!" Behind this kidding was the truth that my wife is the best thing that has ever happened in my life. I often call her my "ordered"—everything that I would want in a woman is in my wife, as if she was made to order for me. My life was as perfect as I could want it to be.

Then, a few years ago, the period that I call My Dark Night of the Soul began. One by one I started losing everything that was— or seemed to be—dear to me. First I lost my health. I sustained a painful injury to my right wrist, which meant I could not work. Then I was diagnosed with prostate cancer and had to undergo surgery. But instead of recovering normally, I developed severe post-surgical infections. One night—it was Christmas Eve—I had a 105-degree fever and felt I was going to die. I required emergency surgery to drain the infection. I survived, but I had raw surgical wounds that lasted for weeks. This left me spiritually, emotion-ally, and physically devastated.

My Dark Night continued. Along with chronic pelvic pain from half a dozen urological surgeries, I developed severe depression. I was on a combination of antidepressants and heavy-duty pain medications. Because I was considered physically well as long as I took the medication, I was deemed well enough to go back to work as an anesthesiologist. But I knew it was not the right thing to do. Even a slight error in my judgment could kill a patient, and with all the medications I was on that slight error seemed very possible. I therefore found myself unable to work, and went on medical disability. I had to sell my house at a substantial loss.

At one point I lost all hope and wanted only to leave this world.

But my wife's steady, true, unconditional love and support prevented me from taking any action to that effect. I can only now imagine how painful it was for her when, on my birthday, I asked for a gift: "If you really love me, please let me go. Life is just too painful." I'm so grateful that she would not give me that "gift" I asked for.

Today I feel that I had to go through all this as a lesson. I had to find my true purpose in life. That's why I'm writing this book. I want to invite you to explore with me what it really means to end pain in all its forms. The keys to that, as I discovered and you will learn, are to forgive, love, and heal yourself. Forgive, love, and heal—and end pain of every kind.

WHAT IS PAIN?

Most of us want our path in life to be predictable, with no rough patches or surprising twists. We are averse to abrupt changes in the path's surface from smooth to rough, sudden hairpin turns and drop offs that mean we have to carefully negotiate ourselves down a bluff to continue our journey. Very simply put, *we want to avoid pain.* Yes, we want to have pleasure, too, but while pleasure is certainly important, it is also secondary. First and foremost, we human beings want to avoid pain. And when pain can't be avoided, we want to get rid of it as quickly as possible.

If pain can be thought of as a "bump in the road," then there are no bump-free roads in life. There are no totally smooth and predictable paths. Sure, most of us find benign sections that are relatively easy to traverse, stretches that allow us to glide along the surface as if we're on roller skates. But sooner or later, there comes the unexpected bend that sets us on a new direction or a difficult expanse that requires us to pay close attention to how we are navigating on our journey.

Regardless of how it may seem at the time, the unforeseen circumstances that crop up as we make our way along our path can be among the most valuable events of our lives. We all know this when we look back on what happened in the past, but somehow current problems always seems much more painful. Well-known examples include the dreaded layoff that eventually leads to another job much better than the first. Or the stressful breakup that frees us to meet the love of our life. Or the unintended pregnancy that seemed devastating and then brings a child that is a priceless blessing.

Even a terrible and painful disease like cancer can be an opportunity for amazing insight and transformation—and I say that as a person who has been a cancer patient. This is not to say that cancer is a good thing. It's just that good can come of it. A *lot* of good can come of it, and that might never have happened if cancer had not swept away distractions and revealed what's really important in every day and every moment.

We can wish that life wasn't so painfully unpredictable and predictably painful. Or we can accept and embrace those circumstances and find ways they can send us in new and possibly enlightening directions. It isn't easy, and it's not supposed to be easy. But here at the start of this book, I want you to know that I'm making these statements from my own severe experience. I have felt my own pain, and I believe that has given me the power to feel yours. But has it really?

When President Clinton said that he felt someone else's pain, how can we understand what he meant by *pain*? It turns out that defining that word is no easy task. It may even be impossible, just as it's impossible to "define" colors like blue or green. We can tell someone how to recognize blue—it's the color of the sky—but we can't directly say what blue is. Pain has a bad name, and deservedly so. Many times I've witnessed the toll that pain can take on a patient, and I've experienced debilitating pain in my own life. In my case the pain was caused by some serious medical issues. But pain can come from any direction—the demands of work, finances, family—or any of dozens of other issues can engender mental and physiological turbulence that can sap our energy and enjoyment of life and threaten our health.

But not everything about pain is bad. The basic physical and mental reactions that characterize acute pain have evolved over the centuries for very beneficial purposes. In the absence of pain, for example, it's difficult to see how children would learn not to burn themselves on the flames of a candle or a match. In fact, there are diseases—one of them is leprosy—in which awareness of pain is disabled, and the effects are very dangerous.

We may experience a version of acute emotional pain at times when we have to give our best performance, such as when taking a driving test or giving a speech. The painful, stress-driven feelings can foster alertness and focused effort.

Another version of pain, however, involves repeated psychologically and physically taxing sensations over a substantial period of time. This happens when pain occurs persistently—when it becomes *chronic*. What makes chronic pain our enemy is that the physiological reactions that characterize acute pain do not stop for days, months, or even years. Because the pain is ongoing, the body doesn't return to its normal state as in the case of acute pain.

Scientific studies have shown that persistent pain is not just a sign or symptom of a specific illness, but also a risk factor for other illnesses. For example, chronic pain can prevent restful sleep. This can contribute to the development of congestive heart failure, which is very often a lethal condition. Chronic pain is also a cause of alcoholism and other addictive behaviors. It can detract from our emotional, social, and spiritual wellbeing, adversely affecting how we get along with others and detracting from the quality of life. It may affect our thinking like a computer virus, creating cognitive blind spots that hide solutions to problems, including the problem of the pain itself.

Considering the importance of pain in human life, it's unfortunate that when medical researchers try to define pain, they quickly hit a wall. The consensus (or the cop out) conclusion seems to be that "pain is whatever someone says it is." Since that's not very use-ful, it may be a step in the right direction to say that pain is any feeling an individual wants to avoid or escape. This includes both physical sensations and emotional experiences. I suggest that it should include spiritual pain, and I will have much more to say about this in the chapters that follow.

Here are some examples of how pain is currently being defined by mainstream medicine. As you read these definitions, you'll see both the strengths and the weaknesses of contemporary health care. There is precise language and careful thought, but there is also a very limited sense of the human dimension of the topic.

- Pain is an unpleasant feeling often caused by intense or damag-ing stimuli, such as stubbing a toe, burning a finger, putting alcohol on a cut, and bumping the "funny bone."

- The widely used definition of the International Association for the Study of Pain states, "Pain is an unpleasant sensory and emotional experience associated with actual or potential tissue damage, or described in terms of such damage."[1]

- Pain motivates an individual to withdraw from damaging situ-ations, to protect a damaged body part while it heals, and to avoid similar experiences in the future. Most pain resolves promptly once the painful stimulus is removed and the body has healed. But sometimes pain persists despite removal of the stimulus and apparent healing of the body, and sometimes pain arises in the absence of any detectable stimulus, damage, or disease.

Despite the fact that pain is very difficult to define, the prob-lem of pain is a tremendously important factor not only in our healthcare system, but in our national life as a whole. Over the course of my career as a physician, I've learned that the majority of patients who seek out health care do so because of pain. Moreover, pain can exist in many forms beyond physical discomfort. If we include emotional pain, not to mention emotional torment, I don't think it's an exaggeration to say that virtually everyone is living with some level of pain. That is what I believe to be true. Literally everyone is trying to live with feelings—physical, mental, emotional, or spiritual—that they would like to avoid or extinguish.

Statistically, it's clear that pain is an immense problem. But what kind of problem is it? As alarming as the numbers are regarding pain as a health issue, one fact is even more startling: Even with the most advanced diagnostic tools, it is often not possible to find and identify the physical cause of pain—and despite treatments of every conceivable kind, many patients continue to have unrelieved pain. Pain is clearly not just a physical problem, so it can't be treated simply by physical means. I can say that with confidence, because I have real-life experience with conventional pain treatments, as both a provider and a recipient.

EMPATHY AND SYMPATHY

We can now see how hard it is to define pain—especially someone else's pain— and we've glimpsed how vast the problem of pain really is. If we return to the Bill Clinton quote, we have to ask ourselves how Clinton could say he feels something without knowing what it really is. In other words, can one person really feel the very intense, very unpleasant, and very individualized sensations in another person's body, mind, and heart?

I believe the answer is both yes and no. But for conventional medicine, the question itself is irrelevant. It's not a doctor's job to "feel your pain." That might be a requirement for the President of the United States, but a physician is trained to look at things in much more objective and material terms. This is probably necessary, and I don't think it's necessarily a bad thing. But it's also very limited in terms of really solving the problem of pain. In any case, there's much to be learned about how pain is assessed and treated by the mainstream healthcare system. It's a model that needs to be greatly expanded, but it provides a good foundation for beginning to talk about pain.

When physicians speak with a patient who is in pain, they naturally begin by asking the patient to describe what the pain feels like. For many people, this is a daunting question and sometimes even an offensive one. Not everyone is gifted with the ability or the vocabulary to talk about his or her pain, especially not while in the midst of it. Still, it can be useful for physicians to hear what patients say, especially if some prompts are offered. "Is the pain dull or sharp?" "Does it come and go, or is it continuous?" "Is it a burning sensation, or does it feel like an electric shock?"

The doctor may next ask about the intensity of the pain. Very often the patient is asked to rate his or her pain on a scale from one to ten. Again, this kind of analysis can be off-putting to someone in severe pain, but it's virtually always part of the initial assessment. It may also have the benefit of getting the patient outside of the subjective experience of the pain, if only for a moment.

By this point the patient will naturally have mentioned the location of the pain, although sometimes this is surprisingly difficult. Many people experience generalized pain that isn't really specific to some part of the body. Others have pain that seems to migrate from one point to another nearby or that appears suddenly in one place and then somewhere else later.

Finally—and I believe this is very important—the doctor may ask about any factors that seem to make the pain better or worse. Often patients will report that pain is worse at night or when they're trying to sleep. Other people wake up with pain in the morning or feel pain as soon as they get out of bed.

Of course, by this time in the assessment people have gotten a very clear message from the doctor. They understand that the doctor wants "just the facts." What's not wanted is an exploration of the emotional crisis the patient might be experiencing that day or (even less welcome) a crisis that happened years before whose effects are still being felt. Sometimes patients will start off in this direction, and most doctors will at least try to listen patiently. But usually it's just a matter of waiting the patient out until the doctor can get back to the real business at hand, which is usually a prescription for pain medication.

While this kind of interview can provide the doctor with essential information from a biomechanical point of view, let me repeat that it has nothing to do with empathy—with trying to feel another person's pain. Anyway, most doctors and most scientists would say that's impossible. There is now some evidence, however, that the human brain is wired to do exactly what seems to have been factored out of accepted medical protocols: It is possible to feel someone else's pain.

This is made possible by a set of brain cells that have come to be called "mirror neurons." These specialized cells were discovered by accident at a laboratory in Parma, Italy, where a group of brain researchers had been working with monkeys. The researchers were testing a neuron—a brain cell—that always fired whenever the monkey would grab for a peanut. As soon as a monkey moved to get a peanut, the neuron would fire. So the scientists believed this was a motor neuron—a cell related to motion.

But one day something very surprising happened. A monkey was sitting perfectly still when he saw one of the researchers pick up a peanut—as he saw this, the neuron fired. Since the monkey hadn't moved—it was the human who moved—it seemed that this particular neuron couldn't tell the difference between seeing something and doing something. The neuron fired in both cases. The implication was that, for this kind of brain cell, watching something happen and making it happen yourself produced the same experience in the brain. Initially these cells were called "monkey see, monkey do" neurons, but that soon changed to "mirror neurons," because through them the brain seems to mirror the movements it sees.

Soon there was an even more remarkable discovery. The researchers learned that mirror neurons can connect us not only with other people's actions, but with their feelings as well. The neurons fired, and fired with a variety of intensities, when human experimental subjects were shown photos of video clips of happy people, sad people, or people who seemed to be in pain. The brains of the observers mirrored the emotional experience of the people who were being observed.[2]

I think you can see why this is so important. When I was practicing medicine, with a specialty in pain management, I naturally felt sympathy for my patients. By sympathy I mean an awareness of what they were feeling, but a conceptual awareness, an awareness from the outside. I saw what they were feeling, and I acknowledged it from an external point of view. That was my training. That was my job. Although not all neuroscientists agree on the significance of mirror neurons, this research does seem to be evidence that one person can feel another's pain. Not just sympathy, but empathy. Not just the President, but anyone. For me personally, this is a very important principle. If I didn't believe it, I would not be writing this book.

2

LIFE AS PAIN OR LIFE AS LOVE?

In light of my professional experience with pain as an anesthesiologist, perhaps it's ironic that I became so personally familiar with pain as well. This included both physical pain as a cancer patient, and psychic pain through my dependency on prescription medications. These were certainly difficult experiences, but I know they're not unique. Millions of people have endured illness, injury, drug dependency, and addiction. We all know how pain *feels*. In this chapter I want to offer some historical and philosophical context to illuminate what pain *means*.

I'll also introduce you to some traditional tools and techniques that people around the world have used to deal with pain. None of them involve drugs, needles, or anything that needs to be plugged into an electric wall socket. They do require some concentration. For example, learning a few basic concepts from the *Bhagavad Gita,* a 5,000-year-old Sanskrit poem, isn't like watching television. But the effort will be well rewarded.

Since the beginning of history the world's great spiritual traditions have tried to confront and understand pain in human life. Not just pain in the body, but also what Shakespeare's Hamlet called "the thousand natural shocks" that can take physical, emotional, and spiritual form.

In the Biblical story of Job, a genuinely righteous man is suddenly subjected to a series of devastating catastrophes. His body is wracked with pain, his family is destroyed, and he loses his home and all his possessions. His friends try to convince him that there must be some good reason for this. Surely God has some worthwhile purpose in mind. But when Job challenges God to explain, God's response is disarmingly simple: "You wouldn't understand." God expresses this in supremely powerful poetic language, but the gist of it is: *You wouldn't understand.*

There isn't much left for Job to do after that except grin and bear it, which is what he tries to do. But there's a happy conclusion. At the very end of the story, Job gets everything back the way it was. Unfortunately, Biblical scholars unanimously agree that the last paragraph of the Book of Job was tacked on many centuries after the original composition. The first draft was a bleak look at the pain of living in an incomprehensible universe. The final text— you could call it the Disney version—sacrifices hard-minded resignation to fill the human need for consolation.

THE ROLE OF AYURVEDA

Western medicine understands pain as a sign or symptom of injury or disease. Disease, in turn, is seen as an abnormal condition, a disorder of the physical structure or the function of an organism. Alternative forms of medicine like Reiki therapy and homoeopathy describe disease in terms of blockages or imbalances of energy that exist in the body.

Ayurveda is a Sanskrit word that refers collectively to the traditional health sciences of India. Since the late 1970s, Ayurveda has gained some recognition in the United States. Today, Americans who are interested in alternative medicine often have at least some knowledge of Ayurveda, and some are genuine experts.

In some ways the position of Ayurveda in America is surprisingly similar to its standing in India, but there are important differences. Regarding Ayurveda, the two countries are mirror images of one another. For example, in the United States interest in traditional Indian medicine is strongest among college graduates and people who are reasonably well off financially. Their level of education allows them to explore unfamiliar terminologies and treatments, and they have money to spend on books, herbs, and other resources. In India, however, in its various forms Ayurveda is much more popular with rural, relatively uneducated people than among the financial elite. It's safe to say that virtually everyone in India has at least heard of Ayurveda, and millions of people use it. But others will have nothing to do with it, just as a portion of the American population will have nothing to do with NASCAR races or smelt fishing.

Differences and similarities between Ayurveda and Western medicine also exist in their views about the relationship between physical health and spiritual enlightenment. In the West, people often begin to eat healthier food after exploring and developing a spiritual practice such as meditation. Spirituality comes first and then translates into a healthier lifestyle. But tradition teaches that Ayurveda developed along opposite lines.

According to legend, Ayurveda originated in ancient times when a group of India's most learned sages gathered in a remote castle. The purpose of the gathering was to create the ultimate system for creating health and assuring long life. But health and longevity were not seen as ends in themselves. The sages believed that the real value of health was that it provided freedom from the pain and suffering that can distract us from spiritual work, which is the true purpose of our lives. In other words, sick people can't develop their souls because they're too preoccupied with their bodies.

As an educated person who earned a degree in Western medicine, I did not see Ayurveda as a legitimately useful approach to dealing with serious illness. I was not uninterested in Ayurveda, though I was fascinated by spirituality and saw a place for it in my life. But when I became ill, I saw both the power and the limits of Western health care. I saw what radiation and drugs could do, and I saw what they could not do and were never intended to do.

For a Western doctor, the purpose of treatment is to return the patient to the same physical condition he or she was in before any symptoms appeared. What happens after that is not really the doctor's concern. For an Ayurvedic healer, what happens after an illness ends is not only a legitimate concern, but it is the healer's most important concern. The highest purpose in Ayurveda is spiritual development. Curing a physical illness is certainly important, but the physical outcome is only a means to a spiritual end.

Once this is understood, it's no surprise that Ayurveda gives even more importance to preventing illness than to curing it. The Ayurvedic sages were aware that once a disease process becomes established, it can be difficult or impossible to eradicate. Consequently, many Ayurvedic teachings involve proper diet, sleep, and exercise.

There is also recognition that the process of disease actually starts long before it can be detected by even the most advanced Western technologies. Yet even at a very early stage, there is always an awareness on the part of the patient that something is not right, that his or her physical system is somehow out of balance. So we must learn to read and act upon the signals sent to us by our bodies. We must sharpen our awareness to a point where it is even more sensitive than an ultrasound or an MRI.

(In this and subsequent chapters, I will introduce Ayurvedic terminology in order to identify concepts specific to this healing tradition. As an author, I feel there is a certain amount of risk involved when I use esoteric terminology. I don't want readers to feel as though you're entering totally unfamiliar territory in which I am the expert and you are merely the beginning student. I think this is an avoidable danger, however, if I offer explanations correctly. Instead of feeling alienated from these concepts, I think you will see them as startlingly recognizable and relevant to your everyday life. The language is different, but the teaching is universal.)

Perhaps the most interesting of all Ayurvedic teachings is the concept of mind/body types. Physically and emotionally, every human being is a combination of three distinct energies, called *doshas*. At birth, these energies are in perfect balance within us— but what is perfect balance for me may be different from what it is for you. Each of us must learn how the *doshas* are proportioned within us. Then we must fine tune our awareness to recognize imbalances as soon as possible. This is an absolutely essential step toward taking responsibility for our physical health, which is the prerequisite for our spiritual development.

During the most difficult times of my illness and treatment, I began to look more closely at Ayurvedic teachings. I was certainly interested in the concept of treating not just symptoms but also causes. The addictions of drinking alcohol or taking drugs are symptoms caused by underlying mental tension or stress. I was also struck by the Ayurvedic idea that toxins can exist not only as viruses or bacteria, but also as ideas and feelings. So nonmaterial toxins produced in the mind or the soul cause symptoms to occur, and chronic pain can be understood as a disturbance of the energy balance in our body.

But the idea of awareness as the first stage of illness was especially meaningful to me. Even when things had been going really well for me, even when I was living the "American Dream" that was so compelling to me, I sensed that something wasn't right. Without trying to look any deeper, I simply paid no attention to that feeling: How could anything be wrong when I had whatever I wanted?

The problem is that sometimes having everything you want prevents you from having—or even realizing—what you need. I'm aware, for example, that it can seem maudlin and sentimental to say we should spend as much time as possible in nature, surrounded by the beauty of forests and mountains. How can that compare to getting a new car every year or flying first class in an airplane? But at the deepest level of our being, we actually do need to be out in nature. We also need good relationships, healthy social activities, feelings of contentment, gratitude, and peace, and, most importantly, we need to give and receive love. I can't prove that with data, but I am convinced these elements help speed the process of healing, which leads to good health, genuine happiness, and freedom from pain in both the body and the soul.

LOVE PROMOTES PHYSICAL HEALTH

There is plenty of anecdotal evidence that positive thoughts and feelings promote physical health. You may have had an experience with this in your own life. Love makes us feel good about ourselves and about others as well. Several studies and research reports have come to the conclusion that love keeps us healthy—or at least feeling healthy—mentally, emotionally, physically, and socially.

Before we start discussing its benefits, we need to first know what love is—a topic I'm sure everybody already has some thoughts about. While every individual might come up with his or her own version of love, I agree with Deborah Anapol, the author of *The Seven Natural Laws of Love*. According to her, love in inherently compassionate, empathic, generous, a free heartfelt feeling without any strings attached, a powerful drive, and a real force of nature that is bigger than us.[1]

Various traditions have categorized many different types of love based on its nature, such as agape, eros, philia, and storge. Every human being has the capability to love any living or nonliving thing. Love can exist between family members, friends, neighbors, co-workers, in addition to the love between amorous partners or couples, which may be our first thought when we think of love. At the level of our daily experience, love is overall a very powerful healing energy that gives meaning to our life, supports us in times of difficulty, delivers strength when we're ill, makes us achieve feats we don't even think of, and may entirely transform a person.

Whatever the form of love, it's quite possible that love has a wide variety of health benefits. We know it really helps to reduce stress, promote mental health, lower the chances of having cancer, lessen pain, improve blood circulation, lower blood pressure, and reduce the risk of heart diseases. It may also help us live longer, and it certainly allows us to live better and feel younger.

When people feel they are experiencing love in whatever form, adrenaline pumps through their bodies. Feelings of love produce the dehydroepiandrosterone (DHEA) hormone, which not only acts as a stress buster but also restores the growth of nerves and thus improves our memory. When we are in love, the release of hormones vasopressin and oxytocin brings a sense of peacefulness and unity.

Studies even suggest that when couples are in love and are happy, they produce less cortisol under stress, leading to lesser negative impact on the immune system. Cortisol is also the culprit responsible for visceral fat stored around the abdominal organs. If one is not in love, stressful conditions produce larger amounts of cortisol, which can lead to diabetes and heart disease. On the other hand, when feelings of affection are expressed this results in lower cholesterol levels, which in turn reduces the chances of suffering a heart attack.[2]

It's science as well as poetry to assert that love strengthens the human heart, and many studies indicate that married people, or those who had confidants, lived longer than those who were single. Love also plays an important part in strengthening the immune system of our body that helps us heal quicker. Love lowers the risk of cognitive impairment, which includes poor mental functioning and memory. Sharing good moments, holding hands, and hugging another person as an expression of love helps the stress associated with heart disease and stroke. Human touch increases production of the hormone oxytocin in the body. Also known as the cuddle hormone, oxytocin has a very simple but very powerful effect: It makes people feel happy and loved.

Love provides a sense of security, fills you with courage, and raises your confidence level—because you know you have a reliable fallback option and trustworthy support. The health benefits of love couldn't be better documented than the review by the Department of Health and Human Services on marriage and health. According to the report, married people in general make fewer visits to doctors, have shorter hospital stays, and thus incur lower healthcare costs than single people without a partner. Unmarried, separated, divorced, or not-in-love men have higher rates of suffering from major depression, suicide, and alcohol or drug abuse.[3]

Not only the couple benefit from the healing effects of love, but even the children experience better physical health in adulthood if they grow up with loving parents. Of course, there are situations in which it's in everyone's best interests for a marriage to end, but it has been my clinical observation that children raised in a two-parent family are less likely to engage in self-destructive behaviors such as smoking and substance abuse. It's simply common sense to infer that families in which all members love each other have a greater probability of being healthy and happy.

The absence of love has been demonstrated to really hurt us physically and mentally. A study by anthropologist Dr. Helen Fisher of Rutgers University observed that the nucleus accumbens region of the brain, which accounts for physical pain, is more active in men and women who describe themselves as "brokenhearted."[4] Failure in love brings on many physical discomforts like back pain, headaches, and diseases, apart from psychological disturbances and mental agony. Those who experience love feel the positive difference in their body and psyche.

With regard to pain, I believe the basic message of what you've just read is very clear. Love counters pain. Where love is, pain isn't. You can't take a love pill or receive an injection of love, but you can allow love to enter your life. It may not happen by itself, and you may have to release some habits that have become deeply ingrained in your being. But opening yourself to love is absolutely worth the effort.

LETTING GO

Once, walking by the ocean at high tide, I felt myself face to face with an infinite sea of consciousness. The waves where huge, but in this apparent chaos of water I saw a deep peace. How ironic: I felt grounded by the water!

I had brought along photographs and other artifacts from my goal-oriented vision board at home—a collage of images, affirmations, hopes, dreams, and desires that I had collected over several years. My children had photoshopped my name on the New York Times Bestseller list, me being interviewed by CNN, me on Oprah, and much more. As I walked, I prayed to Spirit:

"I know not what is good or bad for me, so here I surrender my vision board to you."

Then I placed everything from the vision board in the ocean, and let the tide take it away. As I saw everything disappear, I felt surprisingly joyful and free. My new friend, Yogi Cameron, helped me understand this a short time later. He wrote to me:

"Just know that no goal is necessary, only participation on the path."

In the *Bhagavad Gita*, the god Krishna sets out on the path to live a successful life. The path, he says, is Yoga—which literally means "union."

Union with what? Union with the supreme Self. Not the self who thinks, speaks, and acts, who writes blogs, sets intentions, and creates goal-oriented vision boards. Instead, it's the Self with a capital

S. That Self is much more than the small one concerned with thinking and doing. That Self resides beyond the mind and body and silently witnesses everything we do and everything we are.

In the *Bhagavad Gita*, the divine Krishna says awakening our small self and then living in constant union with this supreme Self is the first step toward success and fulfillment in life. The second step, Krishna says, is taking action, which is expressed by the word *karma*. Although karma has been adopted by people in the West to mean a variety of things, in Sanskrit it simply means "action." The message of the *Gita* is that worldly success lies in taking action only from a state of communion with our higher Self. Any action taken in such a state will be "right action," and its successful completion will be a natural law of the Universe.

This, Krishna tells us in the *Gita*, is the secret of worldly success: "Karma (action) Yoga (union)": action from a place of union with the Higher Self. Success happens essentially in three steps.

1. Establishing Awareness of the Higher Self

There is a dimension of being—and all of us have been there, before our birth, or even before our conception—where there is absolute balance and equilibrium. This is true for every individual human being and also for the Universe as a whole. Both have only potential existence in this primordial state. But once this potential begins to take on material form, the pure state of balance is lost. For inanimate objects—everything from subatomic particles to mountain ranges, from single stars to galaxies—there begins a process of entropy and dissolution. It is an infinitely slow return to the primordial state of formless equilibrium. This process also operates in living beings, of course, in whom the dimension of consciousness also exists. With consciousness comes anxiety, with anxiety comes pain, and with pain comes ego.

Ego is simply that aspect of our being that feels pain. Ego can also feel pleasure, but only as a temporary and ultimately frustrated experience. This is because ego attaches itself to sources of pleasure that by their very nature are lower forms of reality than the primordial, nonmaterial state of balance. Ego, therefore, can be referred to as "the lower self." In contrast to ego, there is also the potential within us to connect with the primordial state. This aspect of our being is "the Higher Self."

2. Learning to Live a Fully Active, Fully Engaged Waking Life While Our Consciousness Remains Wholly Established in and Connected to the Higher Self

Even when ego is at its strongest—or perhaps especially when ego is strongest—most people are at least vaguely aware of another dimension of consciousness. I refer to that dimension as the Higher Self. We may not know what that dimension is, we may not be able to precisely define it, but in each of us there is an intuitive awareness of something beyond the ego-based definition of material success.

Organized religions have come into being to serve this intuitive awareness. The saints, priests, and holy men and women, the rituals and ceremonies, the sacred texts, the exhortations and prohibitions—all of these are expressions of the ego's desire for a higher connection. These tools and techniques work well for many people, but they are not the ultimate solution to our situation as human beings. That solution lies in connection with the Higher Self. The practice of conventional religion will always be fundamentally separate from the Higher Self because the practice of religion involves effort. Effort always takes place on an ego-based level of reality, and that is not where the Higher Self resides. Sometimes the effort built into religion takes the form of deliberately blind acceptance. Believers make an effort to accept and follow the principles and precepts of their religion. This faith may eventually take the form of simply turning off their minds in favor of blind acceptance, or it may involve a continuing struggle against doubt. And sometimes, or many times, doubt eventually wins, which plunges the individual back into the atheistic, materialist existence that religion was created to avoid. The spiritual alternative to this is the delicate balance described in the *Bhagavad Gita:* the ability to live in the physical world while maintaining awareness and connection with the metaphysical Higher Self.

3. Allowing All Our Actions to Arise Only from a State of Union with the Higher Self

The real path to ego-free existence, as well as to worldly success, involves releasing rather than grasping, letting go rather than taking hold. It is a fact, of course, that we live in a material world, and to succeed in that world we need to play by the world's rules. We must educate ourselves, find a place to live, and choose a livelihood. The challenging part, however, is to play by those rules in our daily life while still connecting with the domain of pure balance that exists beyond the material dimension—because it is only in that domain that true peace and bliss reside. We need to take action, but we also need to avoid struggle. We need to survive, but we also need to see how we cannot help but survive at the deepest level of our being. We need to move our life forward in a positive direction, but we must also know that our ultimate purpose is returning to the absolute and effortless state of balance from which we came. We exist at a distance from the Higher Self in our pursuit of success in worldly affairs, but we must also maintain a continuing and unbroken unity with the Higher Self that transcends the meaning of conventional "success."

ESTABLISHED IN YOGA, PERFORM ACTION

In the *Bhagavad Gita,* Krishna says that every action has to be performed with absolutely no attachment to its results. This doesn't mean that we're to refrain from or to suppress action or the desire to act. We can never *not* take action as long as we're living in the physical world. Living itself is a very demanding action. But we must act as if we had no interest, investment, or attachment to what we seek to accomplish by acting. In other words: love freely, give fully, and expect nothing.

> *You have control over action alone, never over its fruits.*
> *Live not for the fruits of actions, nor attach yourself to Inaction.*
> *Established in Yoga [Union], O winner of wealth,*
> *Perform actions having abandoned attachment and*
> *Having become balanced in success or failure,*
> *For Balance of mind is called Yoga.*
> —CHAPTER 2, VERSES 47–48

The secret of success in the physical world, says Krishna, is acting with a dedicated heart all the while expecting nothing—and then letting go completely. It takes a certain kind of mastery to be able to do it. The small thinking, doing, wanting, worrying self struggles deeply with the very concept: If all of me is invested in this, how can I *not* want so badly to see the results of my effort? This is exactly why Krishna says the only way to be able to fully generate success is to operate from a different level altogether—to live and act through Yoga with the Higher Self—because this part of us transcends wanting or needing or agonizing or anticipating and instead is content to simply, silently *be*.

Awareness

My discussion with Yogi Cameron about the *Gita* was perfectly timed. I was deeply mindful of the *Gita* and Krishna's secrets of success one day when I experienced a shift: I had the insight by the ocean, by that sea of consciousness, that whatever my small self may think I desire—and whenever my small self may want it—the entire Universe is not there to deliver me room service just because I have been of pure heart and ask for it. The truth is that the timing and the results of my actions are all out of my control. From somewhere I had the overwhelming awareness that my *ananda* (joy, peace, ultimate completion) is not in the achievement of those outward goals I had set, but instead is in being present to serve, to share, to create, and to contribute. I felt for the first time an immense trust and detachment in leaving the results to Spirit. I can feel that my thinking, waking, being self feels free of the shackles of goal-orientated actions—free of the pressure that I had to somehow get there.

My vision board may be fulfilled, or it may not. I will still do the things I have been doing but without attachment to any fixed desire or outcome. Whatever happens, I am at peace. I am free. It is freedom from a particular goal, freedom from being attached to the results of my actions—but not freedom from the action itself.

It's taken me a long time to move beyond my attachment to my goal-oriented vision board. But I have. I am replacing those outward goals with a new set of values rather than achievements: truth, consciousness, and the divine bliss of the soul.

3

MASKING PAIN

People who are in pain want the pain to stop. That's a very straightforward human reflex. But while the intention to stop pain may be simple, the process of actually stopping it can be difficult and confusing. When drugs are involved, the process can also veer off into dependency and even addiction.

Basically, there are three paths to pain relief. The first path, and the only really successful one, is to eliminate the cause of the pain at its source. The source may be a physical problem. It may also be a hidden emotional issue that can include a spiritual component. In my experience pain includes physical, emotional, and spiritual elements. Dealing effectively with those core issues of pain is the overall subject of this book. Unfortunately, pain is rarely addressed as deeply as it should be in Western medicine and American culture, and I hope to change that. Later in this chapter, I'll have more to say about dealing with the real sources of pain.

PALLIATION AND REPLACEMENT: TWO (UNSUCCESSFUL) WAYS FOR DEALING WITH CHRONIC PAIN

Short of eliminating its genuine underlying sources, people often try to deal with chronic pain in two other ways. One is to cover it up—in medical terminology, to "palliate." This is done with drugs. If you have a headache or toothache, it can be palliated with aspirin or ibuprofen. If they don't do the job, there are prescription drugs such as Vicodin or Percodan. If there is a more serious condition, something that puts you in the hospital, morphine may be used. But palliating pain is only a temporary solution. Sooner or later, the "pall"—from the Latin word *pallium,* meaning cover or cloak—will lift and the pain will return. At that point a stronger dose of the same medicine will be needed or the introduction of a different, more powerful drug altogether.

Another option for pain relief involves replacement rather than palliation. Just as the brain cannot think more than one thought at a time, there are limits to how many contradictory feelings the human body can experience at the same time. High levels of stimulation and excitement can provide transitory relief from physical pain simply because the body can't process everything at once. If someone with back pain tries skydiving, there's a good chance the pain will go away at least for the few minutes it takes to reach the ground. Sometimes people who follow this path can lead extraordinarily productive lives. President Franklin D. Roosevelt, for example, was confined to a wheelchair for most of his adult life due to polio, with all the physical and emotional pain that entailed. But Roosevelt didn't have time to think about his disability while he was leading the country through World War II. In fact, most people in America didn't even know he was disabled, and he himself might have been able to forget about it due to the demands of his office. John F. Kennedy was another president who used hyperactivity to deal with chronic pain. We'll look more closely at the mechanism of pain replacement in Chapter 4.

I have personal experience with both palliation and replacement, just as I have experience with both physical and emotional pain. When I closed my day-trading accounts—and this time I hope the closing is permanent—I had been day-trading stocks on and off for years. Initially I made a lot of money but kept losing it. At one point I closed the account and vowed never to trade again. Then, a few months later, I reopened the account. I used to promise myself that now I would be disciplined. I would follow all the rules, like never putting good money after bad and taking my losses early. I knew all the rules of trading.

But just knowing something is not enough, especially when dealing with an activity that has the potential to become a dependency or addiction. In this sense, for me day trading brought up the same issues as chronic pain and the different ways of dealing with chronic pain.

What Your *Dharma* Has to Do with Chronic Pain

The Sanskrit word *"dharma"* refers to the unique purpose that defines the life of every human being. *Dharma* is what you as an individual are truly meant to do. One person's *dharma* might be playing professional baseball. Another's could be brain surgery or parenthood. I am sure there are people for whom day trading is their true calling in life. I'm also certain that there aren't many of those people, and I am definitely not one of them.

One of our most important tasks in life is to discover our *dharma*. It's not necessarily an easy task to accomplish, and there may be many false starts and distractions along the way. I have since realized that I became involved with day trading because I was in emotional and spiritual pain. At first, this form of gambling served as a cover-up, a palliation, for the pain I was in. Later, it turned into a replacement, an exciting or even euphoric experience as an escape from a painful condition in my soul. Eventually, both these approaches can lead to addiction. I'm not sure I ever really became addicted to day trading—my addiction took a different form—but it certainly was not something that was healthy for me to do. I gave up that habit for good when I took a stock trading book and burnt it in a fire pit. As I did so, I asked the Universe to incinerate this negative habit of mine. I hope I have learned my lesson.

DEPENDENCY AND ADDICTION

When people try to escape from pain, two forms of attempted escape are dependency and addiction. In terms of what we've discussed so far, I characterize dependency as palliation and addiction as a replacement mechanism.

Very often an addiction starts as a dependency. Dependency is a biomechanical experience. It's physical. When the body is dependent, the mind will of course be affected, but the experience has not yet expanded into an all-encompassing lifestyle. It is even possible for a dependency to exist for a prolonged period of time without ever turning into an addiction, although I believe that is rather unusual.

There is no question in my mind that the primary form of dependency in the United States today is dependency on painkillers—and I've chosen that term carefully. Painkillers can come in many forms beside medicines, and throughout this book we'll be discussing those forms and how to deal with them. But even if we adopt a narrower definition that's limited only to medications, this is still the major type of dependency and addiction at the present time.

Proof of what's happening is beginning to appear more often in the media. A 2011 report on ABC News stated:

> It is unclear if Americans are suffering from more pain than ever, but they are definitely getting more prescriptions for it. The use of Vicodin, the most popular pain relief drug in the country, has grown dramatically from 112 million doses prescribed in 2006, to 131 million in the U.S. [in 2011], according to a national survey done by the consulting firm IMS Health. Experts say most of those prescriptions are unnecessary. The United States makes up only 4.6 percent of the world's population, but consumes 80 percent of its opioids—and 99 percent of the world's hydrocodone, the opiate that is in Vicodin.[1]

Along the same lines, here is an excerpt from a Centers for Disease Control report about the prescription painkiller "epidemic":

Deaths from prescription painkillers have reached epidemic levels in the past decade. The number of overdose deaths is now greater than those of deaths from heroin and cocaine combined. A big part of the problem is nonmedical use of prescription painkillers—using drugs without a prescription, or using drugs just for the "high" they cause. In 2010, about 12 million Americans (age 12 or older) reported nonmedical use of prescription painkillers in the past year.

Enough prescription painkillers were prescribed in 2010 to medicate every American adult around-the-clock for a month. Although most of these pills were prescribed for a medical purpose, many ended up in the hands of people who misused or abused them.[2]

As more people get their hands on these potentially dangerous drugs, more are taking them to get high. Dependency is created. When dependency on painkilling drugs is created, the brain is tricked by the neurochemical dopamine, which controls the brain's reward and pleasure centers, among other functions. The body listens to the messages sent by the duped brain and abides by them, leading to dependence. Dependency is a physiological process that, at least initially, is without a psychological or emotional component. Addiction, however, is not just a matter of neural messages and responses. It involves not just the body but also the mind and—in my opinion—the soul as well. True addiction occurs when a person *knows* that something—an activity, a relationship, a drug— will cause harm, but still cannot resist it. In fact, the danger may even be part of the attraction.

ELIMINATING THE CAUSE OF PAIN AT ITS SOURCE: AYURVEDIC PRACTICES

Many books have been written about the phenomenon of addiction and how it takes place. In this book, however, I want to focus less on the development of addiction and more on the solution to it. Can body, mind, and spirit be brought back into harmony to ensure permanent addiction recovery? I believe—I know—that harmony can come about, but it requires getting to the root cause of the pain. It demands a deeper form of experience than palliation or replacement.

Fortunately, there are many ways to access this profound healing. What works for one person may not work for another, and you should feel free to explore all the possibilities. Even in conventional medicine there are treatments that work, although exactly how they work is not understood. You don't have to be a mechanic to start the engine of your car. You just have to turn the key in the ignition. Dealing with pain can work the same way. Find out what works for you, and let the results speak for themselves.

I found my way using a number of alternative practices, but the most powerful was Ayurveda, the Indian system for creating and preserving health introduced in the previous chapter. Ayurveda addresses addiction within the category of *madatya*, literally "intoxication treatment," which is directed toward the cause rather than the symptoms. The addiction—whether drinking alcohol, taking drugs, or any one of a seemingly infinite range of possibilities—is a symptom, whereas the root cause is an underlying mental and emotional imbalance. Symptoms occur because of *toxic residues* produced in the body, mind, and spirit.

To understand what this means, we need to look more closely at the term "toxic residues." This is a fundamental Ayurvedic concept, and there is even a Sanskrit word for it: *ama*, which can be understood as a kind of ash. The sages of Ayurveda used the metaphor of fire (*agni* in Sanskrit) to describe the life functions of a human being—not just the physical activities, but also the emotional and spiritual processes. In body, mind, and spirit, we are designed to thoroughly use up what we take in from our environment. Or if we what we take in is not useful, we are designed to completely eliminate it. But if the *agni* of our being is not burning consistently or efficiently, there will be a residue of *ama* that over time can accumulate and cause damage. This is what's meant by toxic residue.

Ama can exist both mentally and physically. It can manifest as cholesterol in the blood, as phlegm in the throat, or as painfully unresolved memory or anger. In fact, mental *ama* is generally a causative factor in the presence of physical *ama,* since an anxious or depressed person will tend to develop unhealthy lifestyle habits of diet, exercise, or, for that matter, addiction. Therefore, an Ayurvedic path to addiction recovery involves a multistep, holistic approach.

A good time to monitor the presence of both physical and mental *ama* is when you first wake up in the morning. You may notice a thick, sticky substance in your mouth at that time, particularly if you've eaten very rich or fried foods in the previous twenty-four hours. This substance is *ama,* according to Ayurvedic practitioners. Similarly, sometimes you may awaken with your mind burdened with anxiety about the day ahead or, even more likely, with regret about things that happened in the day gone by. This is mental *ama.* It's the kind of sharp regret I used to feel if I lost money trading stocks. Of course, the brief excitement of winning money was a version of mental *ama,* too. Whether it's dejection or euphoria, whether it's mental or physical, *ama* is the residue of unhealthy, self-destructive behavior. If this behavior continues, *ama* will accumulate. Pain will be the result—physical, mental, or both.

The Importance of Diet and Nutrition

At this point there is really no need to introduce the connection between diet and health. Americans have been fully exposed to that concept, even if millions of them continue to behave otherwise. For those who choose or are addicted to self-destructive eating habits, and the pain that comes with those habits, I hope this book will be of value. But I also want to emphasize a point that is not meant to deny the importance of what we eat, but is intended to moderate and refine it.

There is an obvious attraction to believing that whatever is wrong with us can be cured by what we put in our mouths. After all, if we are what we eat, and we are the ones who control what we eat, we should be able to control what we are by means of what we eat. And in extreme cases, diet is definitely the most important factor. If a person is fifty pounds overweight, he or she should definitely stop eating a quart of ice cream every night. But we need to remember that the foundational principle of Ayurveda is *balance*. Someone who deeply enjoys ice cream should not ignore or devalue that enjoyment, but should bring it into balance with other factors. When does ice cream become not just a pleasure but also a risk? By the same token, when does not eating ice cream— or any other food that brings enjoyment— turn into a type of self-denial that can have negative consequences of its own? These are the kind of diet-related questions that everyone needs to ask and answer for themselves.

One general Ayurvedic recommendation regarding nutrition involves herbal therapy. This begins with hot herbal teas and herbal spices in food, with the intention to soothe and balance the digestive system. A diet based on nutritional herbs purifies the body by clearing away the toxins produced in the body, leading to recovery. This could be seen as a form of replacement therapy, with herbal replacement for the experience of pain as well as for the resulting addiction.

A person undergoing addiction recovery should follow a strict vegetarian diet that consists of cooked whole grains, fresh vegetables, and fruits. Such food is highly nutritional and contains all the required vitamins and minerals. A person in recovery from pain or addiction has a damaged nervous system, and he or she requires complete nourishment for total addiction recovery.

Generally, Ayurveda advocates balancing and integrating a variety of foods rather than excluding one or another. It emphasizes the importance of strong digestion, the way specific flavors or tastes balance or don't balance with others, and the danger of using food as a substitute for pleasure or palliative for pain.

Ayurvedic teaching on diet is an enormous topic on which many excellent books have been written. You'll find selected titles in Further Reading at the end of the book.

Yoga and Meditation

Like the connection between diet and health, the once esoteric practices of yoga and meditation have become well-known and widely practiced in the United States. But as with nutrition, I believe there is a tendency to go to extremes. For example, we have mentioned that in Sanskrit yoga means union. One purpose of yoga, and perhaps the most important purpose, is to clarify the connection among body, mind, and spirit. This does not require strenuous yoga poses. It should be energizing and enlightening rather than extreme and exhausting. It is not a competitive sport, despite the fact that yoga may soon become an Olympic event.

Suppose you were to attempt a very simple exercise right now. It doesn't have to be one of the many hundreds of formal yoga postures. It might just be touching your toes (or trying to!). As you do this, you will immediately become aware of certain physical sensations and also certain thoughts and feelings. The exact nature of what you experience will depend on your physical condition and many other factors, but the differences will be a matter of degree rather than basic content. Specifically, you will always notice a certain amount of exertion in order to perform the exercise, and you will always find that making that effort has an effect on the way you are breathing. Finally, if you really focus on what you're doing and try to execute the simple pose in a disciplined and precise manner, you'll also see that you have to concentrate. Your attention will be engaged by the physical action rather than the worries and other static that are always going on in your head.

Of course, the best way to learn about any physical activity is by actually doing it, and toward that end yoga classes are now available in virtually every city and town in America. But whether you're a beginner or a yoga master, the unity of body and mind that yoga clarifies will always be the foundation. It's not about being a contortionist. The slight exertion of the pose, the effect on your breath, and transformation of thought are still the most important purpose.

Meditation is often portrayed as a way to relax, but it's really a powerful tool for feeling more awake and alert. Whether you want to heal from an injury, cure a disease, alleviate stress, find a new hobby, or connect more deeply in your relationships, practicing meditation will help remove blocks to wellness and put you on the path to peace, love, and joy.

There are many forms of meditation. Meditating with a mantra (repeating positive words or phrases that represent qualities you would like to manifest in your life) is one great way to achieve an effective and calming practice. This trains your mind to follow your thoughts and help your subconscious connect with the quality, significance, and energy of those words. Choose any word that resonates with the values that you would like to foster in your life. Or you can use a traditional mantra such as "Om."

To meditate with a mantra, sit comfortably with your eyes closed, and take long slow, deep breaths in and out. Once you feel connected and at ease with the rhythm of your breath, you can begin to chant the mantra as you exhale. Make sure to keep your mind focused on the mantra, and take a slight pause between in-and-out breaths.

Meditating with a mantra is just one option. You can also meditate by listening to the sound of calming music or a guided meditation on CD or DVD. These types of meditation may be easier because you're assisted by the music or the person's voice. This can help you stay focused and relaxed.

Yoga and meditation are really two sides of the same coin. The first purpose of both is awareness. Yoga brings awareness of the connection between mind and body, how carefully executed physical activity can make that connection a closer one. A beginning meditation technique, such as just sitting quietly and paying attention to your breathing, will reveal the mental static that is constantly going on in our heads. The goal of meditation is not to eliminate that static—which is not possible anyway—but to observe it in the same way that yoga students observe the limits of what their bodies are able to do. Both yoga and meditation are very large topics on which outstanding books have been written. Selected titles can be found in Further Reading.

4

REPLACING PAIN

The human mind in some respects has infinite capacity. It's been said many times that most people only use a tiny fraction of their learning capacity, with Albert Einstein often brought up as a notable exception. This may or may not be a scientifically valid observation, but it's very unlikely that anyone has ever learned so much that they're unable to learn anything more. When it comes to absorbing information, the human brain seems to be an endlessly expandable sponge.

In other respects, however, the brain does have definite limits. For example, a human being can only think one thought at a time. If you are thinking of a pink elephant, you cannot at the same moment be thinking of an elephant that's green or blue—nor can you be thinking about a sports car or your income tax return.

Along the same lines, the mind cannot successfully tell itself *not* to think something. A thought cannot be suppressed by another thought. If you tell yourself not to think of a pink elephant, you will necessarily have to think of a pink elephant. There's simply no way around it. Try it yourself.

These principles of thought have counterparts in the physical capacities of the human body. Specifically, the human body cannot experience pain and pleasure at the same time. This fact has important implications for dealing with pain and the problems associated with painkilling drugs. In the previous chapter we discussed ways that pain can be palliated, but *replacing* pain or addiction to painkillers can also be a powerful strategy.

CONVENTIONAL REPLACEMENT THERAPY

When physicians speak of replacement therapy, what they generally have in mind is something very different from what we'll be discussing in this chapter. Replacement therapy usually refers to replacing or counteracting a prescription for one drug for which dependency or addiction has occurred with another drug. There is minimal, if any, focus on emotional or spiritual change in this form of replacement therapy.

There is an enormous market for addiction treatments of all kinds. From a financial point of view conventional replacement therapy has large benefits for pharmaceutical manufacturers. After all, the replacement drugs need to be bought and paid for just like the addictive substances. Millions of people have addiction issues, and many of them will at some point enter treatment.

The basis of conventional replacement therapy is the concept that addiction is a biomechanical disease. The focus is on the chemical changes that addictive drugs bring about in the brain and on ways to impact those chemical changes by using other drugs. Just as a diabetic requires insulin, a drug-dependent person can use a drug to combat the dependency.

Often this kind of replacement therapy is presented as a first step in the recovery process. Once stability has been restored on the biochemical level, the patient will then be able to move toward psychological and even spiritual recovery. But the nonchemical aspects of recovery are really treated as an afterthought, if at all. Fundamentally, addiction and dependency are seen as problems of chemistry rather than soul.

The most common and best known replacement therapy drug is methadone, which is used in connection with heroin addiction. Essentially, methadone creates an effect not unlike the heroin it is supposed to replace. The difference is simply that methadone is "legal" when prescribed by a doctor. Patients often remain on this form of replacement therapy for long periods of time, sometimes for the rest of their lives.

One might ask, therefore, what is the real benefit of methadone treatment or the difference between that and addiction or dependency? Many people would answer "nothing." In fact, for this reason some nations have banned methadone therapy.

A variation of conventional replacement therapy is use of the drug antabuse to combat alcohol abuse. Unlike methadone, antabuse does not mimic the pleasant high of the additive substance. Instead, it produces an extremely unpleasant reaction similar to a very severe hangover. In this way antabuse is intended to "punish" or decondition the user to the point where alcohol is avoided rather than desired.

A DIFFERENT APPROACH TO REPLACEMENT

Given that the human body and the human brain are incapable of experiencing both pleasure and pain at the same time, replacing rather than eliminating pain can be a powerful strategy. This applies to both the pain of a disease or an injury and the pain of an addiction or dependency. But replacement of this kind is not simply a matter of seeking out pleasure. Truly replacing pain requires not just pleasure but real serenity and fulfillment.

According to Ayurvedic teachings, everything in the world—including human thought and consciousness—is comprised of three fundamental elements, called *gunas*. Although the three *gunas* exist in equal measure as potentials or tendencies, they manifest in different proportions depending on the physical health and emotional consciousness of an individual.

Before looking at how the *gunas* express themselves in terms of pain or pleasure, it's important to understand exactly what kind of energy each of the three represents.

1. *Tamas* is usually depicted in negative terms. While it might be tempting to think of the *gunas* as opposed to each other, as good opposed to evil, this would be a mistake. *Tamas* is not "bad" or "wrong." In some ways it parallels the current definition of depression—and no one thinks of depression as evil.

   Tamas is really the energy of no energy, if such a thing is possible. It's inertia, torpor, lethargy, and general lack of vitality. And that's also what depression is. Depression is not intense unhappiness. It's lack of intensity in any form.

   In Ayurvedic teachings, the lack of activity associated with *tamas* is extremely counterproductive for the soul's well-being. After all, the purpose of our being in the world is to work out our karmic destiny and achieve the perfection of our souls. This definitely requires plenty of activity, and *tamas* is the opposite of activity. While *tamas* is not evil, it's certainly not good for helping us achieve the fulfillment of our being or getting rid of pain or addiction.

2. The *guna* called *rajas* can be seen as the opposite, or perhaps the compliment of *tamas*. *Rajas* is identified with energy, motion, and dynamic activity, which is needed to cure pain or addiction.

3. *Sattva*, the third *guna*, is the principle of balance, clarity, and purity. It's more than just the synthesis of *tamas* and *rajas*; it transcends the other two forms of energy. *Sattva* is a condition of steadiness, tranquility, and peace. With respect to life in the physical world, *sattva* involves not only detachment from negativity but detachment from all results of every kind.

These three principles—*tamas, rajas,* and *sattva*—are present throughout creation and in every human life. Management of pain in every form can be understood as replacing or restoring negative, disproportionate aspects of these principles with a more balanced relationship among them. To understand how this takes place with respect to pain and addiction, we need to look more closely at the Ayurveda healing tradition.

Ayurveda, Pain, and Addiction

Pain and addiction related to pain medication are directly related to the brain. Both are at the most basic level simply negative messages sent by the brain to the physical self. Fundamentally, it is the brain that is experiencing an imbalance, and this experience is then transmitted to the body.

Can the brain be brought into the balance and tranquility of *sattva,* and can this become a permanent replacement for pain and addiction? For a certain percentage of people pharmaceutical treatment and rehab facilities can be useful. But more efficient, cost-effective, very powerful approaches are found in Ayurveda and its associated disciplines of yoga and meditation. They provide a holistic, natural, and absolute solution to pain and addiction. By learning to wisely use and fully experience the tools and techniques of Ayurveda, there will no longer be a place for pain in your consciousness. And once there is no place for pain in your consciousness, there will be no place for it in your body either.

Ayurveda exists to treat causes rather than symptoms. Pain, dependency, and addiction in any form are symptoms. The root cause is the stress of underlying mental, emotional, and spiritual imbalance. The symptoms occur in the body because of the toxins or pain produced by the root cause in the mind and spirit.

To expand on Ayurveda's multistep approach introduced in Chapter 3:

1. After you acknowledge the situation and decide to treat it, study Ayurvedic practices and commit yourself to them,

2. Determine the influence of the three *gunas* in your life, as well as imbalances in your mind-body *doshas*, discussed below.

3. Replace your pain with effective remedies to remove the accumulated toxins by following an herbal and nutritious vegetarian diet and establishing a meditation routine and yoga practice.

Identifying Ayurvedic *Doshas* and Using Herbal Remedies

According to Ayurveda, there are three basic psycho-physiological constitutional types called *doshas*. Everyone's experience of life—including the experience of pain and addiction—is influenced by the balance or imbalance of the *doshas* in the individual's mind, body, and spirit.

· *Vata dosha* individuals are characterized by an active nature and sometimes hyperactivity. They are vulnerable to psychosomatic problems and also to addiction to reduce their characteristic anxiety, worry, pain, and insecurity.

· *Pitta dosha* individuals are very energetic and highly focused in their work. When something such as pain or illness causes them to perform less well than they'd like, they may look for chemical solutions to the problem and have difficulty in addiction recovery.

· *Kapha dosha* individuals are a bit lethargic and may become depressed and sedentary when in pain. As a result, they may use addiction for stimulation.

For Ayurvedic treatment of pain and addiction to be effective, the imbalance in the *doshas* needs to be determined, so lifestyle tools and techniques can be defined to normalize them. In my own case, through meditation and by completing a *dosha* and *guna* questionnaire developed by the Chopra Center for Wellbeing in

Carlsbad, California (doshaquiz.chopra.com), I discovered I was *pitta* imbalanced. So I started to follow a *pitta* pacifying diet and also take the appropriate herbs, such as amla, ashwagandha, shatavari, and bhramari. These and other herbs and herbal preparations are available online at ayurvedicbazaar.com/rasayanas.php.

Herbal therapy begins with hot herbal teas and herbal spices in food, which are intended to soothe and balance the battered digestive system. This is fundamentally a form of replacement therapy, with herbal replacement for the experience of pain as well as for the resulting addiction. A diet based on nutritional herbs purifies the body by clearing away the toxins produced in the body, leading to recovery.

The person seeking recovery starts with a damaged nervous system and requires complete nourishment for total addiction recovery. That person needs to follow a strict vegetarian diet that consists of cooked whole grains, fresh vegetables, and fruits. Such food is highly nutritional and contains all the required vitamins and minerals. The diet should also include ghee (clarified butter), which acts as a lubricant and gives strength to the immune system.

"SOFTWARE FOR THE SOUL"

As part of my recovery process, I attended the Meditation Teacher Training program at the Chopra Center where I became certified to teach Primordial Sound Meditation. While I was at the world-renowned center, I attended a talk by its founder, Deepak Chopra, M.D., one of my role models. Someone in the audience asked him: "Deepak, why did you start to meditate?"

His answer was simple: "Because I wanted to quit smoking and drinking. It was many years ago." He went on to explain a concept that has fascinated and compelled me with its brilliance—the concept of the "software of the soul." We all know about software that runs our computers, our smart phones. We are forever downloading updates or being automatically updated, improving our software to improve the processing time and performance of our machines. But we rarely think of "software of the soul," the operating system that runs the apparatus of our mind and body. Dr. Chopra described it as having three main components:

1. Action: *karma* in Sanskrit

2. Memories: *samskara* in Sanskrit

3. Desires: *vasansa* in Sanskrit

They form a loop so that:

· Action leads to memories.

· Memories lead to desires.

· Desires lead to further action.

Dr. Chopra explained, "It's as if one is on a karmic hamster's wheel." It struck me that this concept applies to all our actions, whether they are apparently simple, harmless actions or whether they are life-destroying actions like addictions.

Here are some examples:

Action to Memory. Eating a piece of chocolate creates a memory. Eating chocolate tastes really good, it's sweet, and we experience temporary relief thanks to the sweetness of the taste!

Memory to Desire: This creates a desire: Next time I am lacking sweetness in my life, I will remember that I can get sweetness from chocolate and that will make me desire chocolate!

Desire to Action: The desire for some sweetness for temporary relief from study or work, stress, or fatigue will lead to the action of going to the store and buying some chocolate or taking some out of my stash in the cupboard.

Another example related to addiction:

Action to Memory: When a person is feeling low, drinking alcohol makes him or her feel better, and it very temporarily relieves the deep emotional pain that disturbs, confuses, and produces anxiety.

Memory to Desire: When the person is feeling the discomfort of anxiety, confusion, or suffering, he or she has a memory that all of this can be quickly relieved by alcohol.

Desire to Action: Now the need to relieve the discomfort is so intense that the person must have alcohol. Relief is sought above and beyond anything else. The person is driven to drink and becomes an alcoholic.

In my own experience, the sequence proceeded like this:

Action to Memory: When I felt low from physical or emotional pain, taking prescription painkillers made me feel better temporarily.

Memory to Desire: Subsequently, I drew on the memory that immediate relief was available from painkillers.

Desire to Action: Therefore I sought and took painkillers.

Unfortunately, this karmic wheel may continue and keep getting progressively worse and injurious, no matter what cost the person has to pay in terms of relationships, jobs, health, shame at being overweight or arrested for drunk driving, and even in extreme cases isolation due to social disrepute. This is the life of the addict, a slave to memories, desires, and actions, as if he or she had no option but to run around the karmic wheel.

But there is a way to get off the karmic wheel, as Dr. Chopra explained, by upgrading the software of our soul. How can this be accomplished? Let's look at a revised version of the karmic sequence for the alcoholic.

Action to Memory: Through the practice of meditation, the person addicted to alcohol often gets glimpses of expanded consciousness, of pure potentiality and pure bliss. This creates a memory of higher states of awareness that he or she will seek out again. That might inspire the person to volunteer at a homeless shelter, which creates a new memory at the soul level and in the mind and body. Serving others removes the focus on his or her own discomfort. Research has shown that by helping others our body responds by decreasing levels of harmful stress hormones and elevating happy molecules like oxytocin, endorphins, and the release of cellular regenerative growth hormones.

Memory to Desire: The next time when the need to relieve anxiety, discomfort, pain, or sadness arises, the person remembers that feeling good comes from meditation and from being in service to others. Those memories lead to the new desire to seek relief through meditation and service to others rather than to alcohol.

Desire to Action: The need to feel good will be followed by taking action through meditation and selfless service to others, and thus the vicious circle of addiction is replaced by positive, life-affirming action. The person will feel infinitely better, make nourishing choices that support his or her ability to be responsible to family, job, and society, and in the process, those even more needy are being supported and helped.

I believe that improving or upgrading the software of our soul is a very powerful concept and a very practical way to replace the pain of addiction.

PART TWO

THE PROCESS OF PAIN

Every religion, every spiritual tradition, and perhaps even every government or political system must confront a single, all-important question: Why do innocent people suffer? Or as the title of an all-time best-selling book puts it: "Why do bad things happen to good people?"

In the next three chapters we'll address the question of "bad things" happening the pain they cause and the ways of dealing with that pain at all levels of our being.

5

CRISIS

We all have experiences that bring the question of human suffering directly into our lives. If we try to integrate the experience with the idea of God as described in the major Western religions, there is no way to avoid a very challenging conclusion: Either God is not all-powerful, or God is not all good. Fortunately, we don't have to come to a conclusion about the nature of God in order to face what philosophers call "the problem of evil." While there's no doubt that this problem can cause a great deal of pain, we can also be certain that the pain can be faced and eventually healed.

Why?

A while ago my twenty-one-year-old nephew was killed in a tragic car accident. Considering the way it happened, it's hard not to think some invisible evil force was planning it. But even if there were such a force, that might be easier to accept than the idea that extremely painful experiences simply happen at random, as if by a roll of the dice.

My nephew had just graduated from a prestigious university in Singapore. He was to begin his first job on Monday, but on

Saturday he died. The pain of my sister and her husband was unimaginable and almost unbearable to witness.

But a crisis in life must be witnessed, and that's only the beginning. We must have the courage to fully experience even the most difficult circumstances and the pain they cause. Nothing can be sugar-coated. The crisis will continue until it has been recognized, solved, and then resolved. The process of making that happen will be the subject of this chapter and the two that follow.

Seeing and feeling this death so closely was like an earthquake in my consciousness. My inner self, the core of my being, was displaced and repositioned. I learned the meaning and value of the present moment—of *now*—and this brought me to a profoundly different state of being.

I am not saying that this is the first time anyone has been killed in an accident; such accidents have happened before and continue to happen. But when it is personal, the pain is very transformative. We are suddenly challenged to let go of our mental chatter from the past and our worries about the future, to look beyond the material dimension of our lives and the world around us in order to connect with a higher reality. But how can we look beyond the crisis of a senseless tragedy and the pain it brings?

MAYA, THE GODDESS OF GREAT ILLUSION

The material dimension of our lives is expressed by the Sanskrit word *maya*. It's a word that has many layers of meaning and association, but they are all tied to the material environment in which we live and with which we can become preoccupied or even obsessed.

I have been thinking a lot about *maya*. I've been inspired to think about it because of something that took place at the Chopra Center in California, where I was earning certification as a meditation instructor. Toward the end of my stay, I was one of at least 300 people who attended a lecture by Dr. Deepak Chopra, who is truly one of my favorite teachers. During the lecture the topic of *maya* came up, which he referred to as "the Goddess of Great Illusion."

I was sitting in the back of the room, far away from the stage. I was completely taken by surprise when, in the middle of educating the audience on the topic of *maya,* Dr. Chopra paused and addressed me personally in Hindi,

"Rajiv ji, do you hear me? Are you understanding this?"

I was shocked that he even knew I was in the room. Why was he addressing me directly in Hindi! Probably no one else in the room could even understand what he said. What must they have thought? I found myself declaring an instant reply:

"Yes, sir!"

In the following weeks, I wondered why Dr. Chopra had singled me out about whether I understood what *maya* is—about what causes us to confuse illusion and reality. After deep refection and meditation, I got the answer.

Maya can most simply be defined as the concept of illusion, based on the principle that our everyday experience and indeed all material reality is an illusion. It's the view that the material world—including our bodies and our minds—are just tricks that delude us from the true nature of ultimate reality that we and the entire Universe are One.

The *Bhagavad Gita* teaches that it's an illusion to think that there is a Cosmic Creator that is separate from you or me. The truth is that you and I are manifestations of that Cosmic Creator. We are not creations of something that is separate from ourselves. We are expressions of a collective energy in a particular form, but fundamentally we are still One with that energy.

You are part of that collective energy. So am I.

If we could just see the larger truth, we'd understand that there is only one reality. The multiplicity of experience, identity, and individuality are not actually real: They are just illusions of separateness. This is what it means to experience *maya*—the illusion of separateness.

Living in the illusion of our self as limited to a physical body, we become very attached to our experiences—seeking better and better feeling ones, avoiding those that would give us discomfort. We begin to pursue things that we decide it would be nice to experience or to have: possessions, positions, power, fame, wealth. We develop desires and aversions. We become so attached to our physical experiences that we forget who we are and what we need to do in order to be our real selves in the largest sense. We become so very attached to our actions, believing that we must achieve what we want on the material level and pursuing every avenue open to us for success. All the while we believe that we are the initiators of our actions. But this is not true. The truth is we are not the "doers" of what we do. *Maya* is.

We are sleepers pursuing a dream that we think is real. Our own divine identities are witnessing our ignorance in the background, waiting for us to wake up.

I understand now that Dr. Chopra was reminding me where freedom from pain and true fulfillment can be found. Finding them depends on making conscious choices that are authentically enlightened. When we become aware of the presence of *maya* in our lives, we can begin to make our decisions in the light rather than in the dark.

Enlightened choices happen from an awareness of true reality and the true self. In other words, they happen when *maya* has been transcended. And *maya* is transcended by the practice of detachment—which is not an easy concept to understand, nor to practice. In the *Bhagavad Gita,* the god Krishna explains it like this: "Anchored in spirit, take action in the material world." In other words, we must grasp the fact that the world of our senses is an illusion, but we must still participate in it to the best of our ability. We must understand that life is essentially a game in which a huge element of chance exists, but we must still try to play the game as well as we can. Trying to withdraw from the game is not really an option, because the game is all-encompassing. The game includes even the act of trying to withdraw from it.

Dr. Chopra was reminding me to make choices from higher awareness, from the *Bhagavad Gita* principle: "Anchored in spirit, take action in the material world." For example, I am writing this book because I want people to read it, but every word I write may or may not be read. Every idea I offer may resonate with many people or with none. My thoughts and my actions need to be anchored in spiritual realization. That anchoring is my responsibility and is within my control. The material results are not in my control. They will be as they will be.

The great poet Rumi said: "When you do things from your soul, you feel a river moving in you, a river of joy." There is truly nothing to achieve but to serve and share, and these acts take one beyond happiness toward a true bliss. After my very public "private" comment from Dr. Chopra, I now feel liberated and free—because the experience caused me to focus on what my motivation is. To reflect on whom I want to be and who I really am.

APPRECIATING THE VALUE OF NOW

I hope no one ever experiences a tragic situation like the death of a young family member. But I also know that many people will face something like that in their lives. Perhaps, even from tragedy, we can learn to appreciate the value of *now*. As Eckhart Tolle has written in his book *The Power of Now,* "Life is now. There was never a time when your life was not now, nor will there ever be."

Perhaps we can learn this not only from our own experiences but from what happens to others. A proverb states, "Life is but writing on sand which we know not when the ocean waves will erase." This puts me in mind of an ancient Indian spiritual text, the *Katha Upanishad*, which is a dialogue between *Yama*, the god of death, and *Nachiketa*, a small child.

In the text, *Yama* is impressed by the sweetness of the boy and offers the child three wishes. For his third wish *Nachiketa* asks to be taught the mysteries of what lies after death. The god of death is reluctant and suggests the child ask for something else—something more material, more tangible, more immediately enjoyable.

Nachiketa won't agree. He asks how anyone who has come close to death can ever again ask for material comforts. Having faced the certainty that all material pleasures will be over sooner or later, one's perspective naturally shifts. When he has encountered death, how can he ask for wealth?

In return for his impassioned and sincere inquiry, *Nachiketa* is taught self- knowledge. He is shown that there is a dimension to being that is beyond the body, beyond every sensation the body allows us to experience. He discovers that the human soul is the true self—and this self is separate from the body.

To live fully is to know that alongside the material triumphs and pleasures our physical selves experience and value, we actually live more fully when we value and cherish the awareness that there is an aspect to our being human that is beyond the physical self. There is a "soul self" that we can each realize and experience.

Easier Said Than Done?

While I fully believe everything I've written so far in this chapter, I also know—both as a physician and as a patient—that the philosophy of detachment can be difficult to practice in times of crisis. So it's important to look at explicitly practical approaches to dealing with this pain. Once you've regained a solid emotional foundation, it will be much easier to achieve a perspective that will allow you to detach from the urgency and turmoil of the crisis.

During World War II, a British psychiatrist named John Bowlby worked with children who had become separated from their parents. When the major cities of England were being bombed every night, a decision was made to move large numbers of children to safer areas of the country, even though this meant breaking up families for a period of time. This was certainly a crisis period for everyone involved, and Bowlby was able to develop valuable information about the dynamics of extreme emotional pain. He also contributed to our understanding of grief through his work with dying children and their parents. Though difficult, this material provided extremely valuable insights that Bowlby presented in three books entitled *Attachment, Separation,* and *Loss.*

John Bowlby identified a series of stages for dealing effectively with a life crisis. They are not a simple progression, and people often go back and forth between one stage and another before finally moving forward.

1. *Shock and Numbness.* In any crisis, the sudden pain can cause the body and mind to function less efficiently, or even to shut down in some respects. This might even be a kind of survival mechanism, since the pain might be too much to bear if a normal level of sensitivity was maintained. There may be difficulty with concentration, impaired judgment and decision making, and a general inability to function normally.

2. *Yearning and Searching.* This includes such wide ranging emotions as guilt and anger, yearning for better days in the past, and painful wondering about the meaning of life and loss. There may be a tendency to withdraw from other people, even close family members, which may continue for a substantial period of time.

3. *Disorientation and Disorganization.* In this phase the sense of pain and loss can seem overwhelming, as if it were the only reality. The rest of life can seem unimportant or even unreal.

4. *Reorganization and Resolution.* Gradually, from the depression of the previous stages, energy returns along with the ability to feel joy again. This is the time when we can begin to look at what took place with some understanding and perhaps a degree of wisdom.

The timeframe for passing through these stages will clearly vary from one person to another. The initial response to crisis is shock, emotional numbing, and disbelief. Usually in a few days this turns to agitation, wishing that things were different, and remembering better days. For most people, agitation and emotional pain are worst around two weeks into the crisis. This is followed by depressive symptoms, which peak about a month later. Sharp feelings of grief can still happen at any time, sparked by people, places, or things. For most people, the whole process of recovery from the pain of a major crisis takes from one to two years.

What Not to Say

A crisis such as the death or illness of a family member is never the experience of just one person. It's a shared situation, and this can be the key to finally bringing about healing. But this doesn't happen by itself. Everyone tries to say the right thing and share the appropriate feelings, but a grieving person will often believe that only he or she really feels it deeply and intensely.

So what should you say or do for those close to you during a painful, highly emotional crisis? It's difficult to know. But there are certain things you shouldn't say:

- "I know how you feel." No one can really know how another person feels. Saying this during a crisis may be well intentioned, but a person in pain may experience it as dishonest.

- "It is God's will." This just raises the problem of how a benevolent God could possibly "will" the terrible things that happen in people's lives.

- "Everything happens for a reason." Even if this is true, it's not much comfort if we can't possibly imagine what the reason might be. What's more, even the most negative and dangerous people think their actions are justified by a good reason. This is of no comfort to the victims of their actions.

Rather than any of the above responses, just saying, "I'm sorry," can mean so much to a person in crisis. It may also be helpful to encourage a person to show the grief and pain they're in, since many people try to hold back. Offering practical help is also important. People in deep crisis can't be expected to deal effectively with the everyday demands of life. Offering to prepare meals, buy groceries, and help with child care can be very positive. It's even better if this help can continue for a significant period of time. People who have lost a loved one—or who are sick, injured, or in pain themselves—will need not days, but months or years to recover.

Living in the Now

In my own life and from my own close encounter with death, I have been taught—just like the small *Nachiketa* in the fable—to give up any attachment to the past or anticipation of tomorrow. I seek instead to live fully and to live only in the now. This present moment awareness is also a form of mindfulness meditation. Here are some practical tips for living with present moment awareness:

1. Be completely here. Don't be distracted by thoughts of the past or the future. The present moment is actually the only real thing there ever is. Give yourself fully to this moment in time.

2. Be thankful for what you have. Try not to regret what you once had or think about what you will have. The past is passed, and nobody knows what the future brings.

3. Do not go to your death with your song still unsung.

4. Or have regrets of not saying "I love you" to somebody.

5. Live every day to the fullest as if it is the last day of your life.

6. Hold no grudges. Forgive, love, heal.

7. Have gratitude for life as it is; start a gratitude journal.

8. Honor the past. Learn from it. But do not dwell in it.

9. Similarly plan for the future, but do not live in it.

10.   Practice love and compassion *now*, especially for those less fortunate than you.

In the chapter that follows we'll look further at moving from the pain of a crisis to a solution. We'll also see that solution is not the same as resolution, which is ultimately the only permanent answer to pain.

6

ADJUSTMENT

In order for the human race to survive, the human form has had to continuously adjust. We as a species have experienced an evolution of the physical body. But the importance of our evolution now extends beyond ourselves. Human survival today is not just about human beings, but involves the survival of the world environment. We must be flexible. We must adjust—and we must have the courage to do so. This does not require changes in people's physical characteristics, but in the evolution of people's consciousness.

What does "evolution in consciousness" mean? It begins with understanding the true nature of thought. Every thought starts with a desire, which may or may not get fulfilled. But that's only the beginning. The actions we take to fulfill our desires, and more importantly how we react when the desires are fulfilled or not fulfilled, express the current level of evolution in our consciousness.

LEVELS OF DESIRE

Let me describe this in a systematic way. The conscious levels of desire can be categorized as follows:

61

The lowest level of desire. These desires arise from physical need, the lowest level of awareness. This does not mean that physical needs are "lower" in any moral or ethical sense. It simply means that this level of desire is based on biological processes. An example would be the desire of an addict to get his or her substance of abuse. Addicts are ready to go to any lengths whatsoever to fulfill that need. It could involve breaking the law, stealing, not caring for others feelings, or not caring for how it affects not only others but also themselves. A related impulse could be the desire to advance materialistically, to make money at any cost: to lie, deceive, and trample on others. The strange thing is the way this is not only tolerated, but actually celebrated by Western culture. Why does a society ennoble such obviously antisocial behavior?

The second level of desire. Here a person has a desire for a goal in a somewhat higher level of consciousness. It's no longer just a matter of desire as a base physical function. More emotion and spirit are involved. If these desires are fulfilled, the person is very happy. If the desires are not fulfilled, the person is angry, depressed, very possibly aggressive, and even physically or emotionally dangerous.

Consider, for example, a person who has an intense desire to be rich. Such a person may begin by working very hard and in an ethical manner, not stealing, robbing, or ignoring the needs of others. If the desire or goal is met, the person is elated. But if it is not met, what happens? The desire for material success can override ethical considerations. "Whatever it takes" becomes the person's mantra, the magic word or words that will cause the object of desire to materialize. And if the desire is still not met, the person can become so angry, frustrated, or depressed that this leads to other self-destructive behavior such as addiction, alcoholism, or becoming short tempered.

Either way, desire at this level—and the "success" or "failure" that results—is almost always an extreme experience of either elation or disappointment. The German social philosopher Max

Weber made the point that as modern industrialized society came into being, the emotional energy that had previously been attached to getting into heaven was transferred into a desire to get rich. Along with this, the faith in God's miracles became faith in the material power of science and industry. This didn't solve the emotional problems that existed in a strictly religious society; it just substituted a new set of anxieties. Where people used to become depressed at the possibility that they were sinners and might go to hell, now they faced the stress that they could end up as low-income losers.

The third level of desire. Spiritually, this is a dramatically higher level of human evolution. Here the person has desires and goals, works hard to fulfill them ethically, but reacts to whether they are fulfilled or not in a less dramatic way. There's an awareness of something beyond the simply material experience of existence. It's not the traditional afterlife of heaven with harps and pearly gates. It's more abstract, or even transcendent.

A person operating from this level begins to experience a spirit of surrender to a divine spirit. It's not that the person doesn't care about whether there is material success or failure, but the person is able to detach from the outcome once the action has been taken. This results in an evolving, higher level of consciousness. As it is written in the *Bhagavad Gita:*

> *"To action alone hast thou a right and never at all to its fruits; let not the fruits of action be thy motive."*
> —CHAPTER 2, VERSE 47

The highest form of desire. This is rarely seen in the modern era, and perhaps it has always been rare. We tend to imagine that in the past there were more spiritually evolved individuals walking around in the world, but I tend to doubt this. After all, when survival was a constant concern—even in terms of avoiding starvation—it's not realistic to think that people were inclined toward saintly behavior. The truth is, if there was ever a time when human beings had a real opportunity to lead highly evolved spiritual lives, that time is now.

In the highest level of desire, a person functions from the ultimate level of expanded consciousness. He or she is almost without desire with respect to personal gains or material advancement. It's all about sharing and service, with higher consciousness expressed at every moment. This is the level in which Buddha, Krishna, and Christ lived and acted. They still went about their daily lives but from a level of true enlightenment.

Meditation and the Evolution of Desire Consciousness

At the very least, meditation is a process of mental adjustment. It's a tool for shifting away from one form of thought into another. With practice, it can become much more. It can bring about genuine transformation not just of thought, but also of emotion and spirit. Although that level of transformation may not happen for everyone, meditation can still be an extremely helpful and useful activity. Even if you never become a concert pianist, learning to play the piano can still be a worthwhile thing to do.

As you are aware, meditation is a state of being that's often associated with Eastern spiritual traditions, especially Hinduism and Buddhism, but it has also been practiced in various forms in Western spiritual traditions. In modern biomechanical terms, it has earned the definition as one of the four states of existence. The other three are wakefulness, sleep, and dreaming.

One beauty of meditation is that a person does not have to be religious or spiritual to take advantage of its practice. Its benefits can be divided into physical, mental, and spiritual.

There are many physical benefits of meditation, which have been known since ancient times. However, they have become better known in the West since the 1960s when meditation, as it is now practiced, was brought to the West by spiritual leaders such as Maharishi Mahesh Yogi of Transcendental Meditation fame. In addition, research by various Western universities using lab studies and modern-day instruments such as the EEG (electroencephalogram) and brain-scanning equipment have helped bring these benefits to light.

Multiple physiological benefits have been discovered with current technologies. The meditative state has been found to elicit the "relaxation response," a term coined by Herbert Benson, M.D. of Harvard Medical School. It is also known as the "rest-and-repair" state. The relaxation response is the opposite of the "fight-or-flight response," which is a necessary reaction found in both humans and lower animals when faced with danger.

In the fight-or-flight response, the sympathetic nervous system goes into overdrive to help the organism survive the danger. The response consists of various physiological changes that take place through the activities of neurotransmitters and the emission of certain hormones. As a result, heart rate, blood pressure, and glucose consumption increase, and a heightened mental state occurs as the animal prepares, in the face of the danger, to fight or to take flight.

Though the fight-or-flight response is common to both animals and humans, there are important differences. For one thing, after the danger passes, the animal goes back to normal baseline. An example often seen on television is a gazelle who, when faced with a lion, goes into this hyper state and runs for its life. But a few minutes later, when the danger has passed, the gazelle is grazing calmly as if there had been no danger at all.

In contrast to the gazelle's behavior, when we humans enter the hyper state, we continue to live in that state for long periods. This is largely because humans often perceive a much wider range of possible dangers than animals, and these perceptions continue for long periods of time. For example, humans may enter the hyper state simply from perceiving threats in such areas as relationships, finances, work, personal efficacy, and future success. Faced with such concerns, we may feel threatened virtually all the time. This can result in chronic stress and various stress-related physical ailments such as heart disease, stroke, and diabetes. These ailments are partly related to the effects of abnormally stress-heightened levels of hormones such as epinephrine, cortisol, and ACTH (adrenocorticotropic hormone).

A major physiological benefit of the regular practice of meditation is that it helps bring hormone levels back to their baseline and thereby helps to heal some modern-day stress-related ailments. Chronic stress can have adverse psychological effects, including depression. In addition, various addictions may arise. To compensate for continual stress, the individual may seek relief through mind-altering chemicals such as alcohol, narcotics, or other drugs.

The effects of meditation on the brain can be measured in modern laboratories. Under the influence of meditation, the hyperactive brain calms down, as is shown by reduced red areas on PET (positron emission tomography) scans. On an EEG, the so-called brain cardiogram, β (beta) waves that represent the hyper state are replaced with slow Δ (delta) waves. That's why meditation has become a part of modern addiction programs. By counteracting the physiological effects of stress, there is less need for the individual to seek out chemicals to alleviate stress.

The rest-and-repair state brought about by meditation helps calm the mind and emotions and often instills a sense of serenity in the practitioner. Meditation helps heal psychological trauma, be it from childhood, post-traumatic stress syndrome, or other sources. It does this partly by helping the individual put events, issues, and concerns into perspective and by substituting a freer-flowing style of thinking for the more analytic thinking that accompanies and stir up anxieties.

Spiritual benefits of meditation certainly exist as well, although there are no instruments to measure those effects. Meditation as a spiritual path has been practiced since ancient times. Often, repetition of various mantras, representing various aspects of God, is a commonly practiced form of meditation.

Meditation in the spiritual sense can be viewed as a means for communing with a higher reality, whether that is called God, our Higher Self, or the all-pervading life force of Hindu belief referred to as *Prana*. This experience of communion or connection allows the practitioner to grow from the outside-in, leading to serenity and gratitude for life itself.

Meditation as a path to God has been known by various names in Eastern culture, including *Dyan Yoga* and *Janan Yoga*. The term "yoga" in this sense means union with our True Nature or God, and thus goes far beyond various stretching exercises and postures.

Meditation can take us to the so-called "gap state" as defined by the Wayne Dyer, one of the founders of the current wave of interest in spirituality that began in the 1970s. As Dyers explains, meditation takes us to the gap between our thoughts where there is nothing. It thereby connects us to the universal "black hole" from which, according to some, the whole universe came into existence.[1] According to some Eastern traditions, this nothingness is the formlessness that gives rise to the forms that constitute the reality that we perceive through our senses.

Meditation as a spiritual exercise can also be viewed as helping us connect with a supreme, all-pervasive intelligence, a divine creative consciousness. This connection might then lead to a "breakthrough" experience in which the Divine manifests itself through a wonderful new piece of music, art, writing, or some other achievement.

SEVA: THE POWER OF DESIRE BEYOND DESIRE FOR OURSELVES

Nowadays, the Sanskrit words *karma, mantra, pundit, dosha,* and *chakra* have become mainstream. There is one such word, however, that is not as well known but needs to be. The word is *seva,* which in Sanskrit means "service."

Seva is not just any kind of service, but rather selfless service performed with a sense of gratitude, as we discussed in Chapter 4. It is service infused with kindness and respect for the ones served, and it gives rise to peace and love. It is an act of mental and emotional adjustment in a direction *away* from ourselves and our individual needs *toward* the needs of others and of humanity as a whole.

If we all were to do our work and carry out our relationships in accordance with *seva,* the world would change profoundly. *Seva* is not about taking a few hours out of our busy week to help others. It's not something to be turned on and off, as if kindness, compassion, and gratitude are qualities to be doled out in limited amounts. *Seva* is about designing our lives in such a way that we consistently serve others selflessly. Every action, every interaction should be *seva.* This includes in our work lives.

Professionals of every stripe—lawyers, doctors, dentists, and others—often assume a distant or even superior attitude toward their clients or patients. They fail to connect with the other person's humanity. For caregivers to have such an attitude is especially sad because for such professions, the rewards of *seva* are great. If a doctor, for example, greets a patient with an attitude of compassionate service, with actions and words that essentially say, "I am thankful to you for finding me worthy of service to you, and for providing the means of my livelihood," then the doctor will likely find that the patient already feels better before anything else is said or done.

Seva is not selective. It does not evaluate our fellow beings and choose some for care and respect while ignoring others. It treats all humans with compassion and tenderness. As a Taoist verse says, "I work at eliminating all my judgment of others."

Taking up an attitude of service with gratitude provides us with many rewards in all four dimensions of our lives: physiological, social, mental, and spiritual.

In regard to physical pain, *seva* is a source of positive energy, which Professor Barbara Frederickson of the University of North Carolina reports is linked to a number of physiological benefits. These include a decrease in stress hormones, lowered blood pressure, and improved immune system functioning. Practicing selfless service with gratitude also increases our levels of the feel-good hormones prolactin and DHEA (dehydoepiandrosterone).[2]

Socially, to practice seva is to recognize the natural bond between ourselves and others. When we let *seva* guide our interactions with others, we create open spaces where people feel acknowledged, respected, and cared for as their barriers come down. Kindness and compassion take us out of our selfish egos and expand us, making us larger. We strengthen our relationships and friendships, while creating new ones. Socially, everyone benefits from *seva.*

Mentally and spiritually, *seva* promotes powerful happiness-creating emotions—kindness, caring, and gratitude. This not only brings profound karmic benefits, it infuses our lives with meaning and value, lifting us up spiritually along with those we serve. By profoundly affecting all four of our dimensions, seva builds health, peace, harmony, and joy in our lives.

We can even take *seva* into the bedroom with us. Sex without *seva* is just sex. But when this basic natural act is approached as *seva,* it becomes lovemaking. With *seva,* you do not simply aim for your own personal satisfaction. Instead, you focus on pleasing your partner, giving all you can to making her or him happy. Your partner's response to this selfless attitude then creates delight for both of you. What results is a wonderful mix of physicality, psychology, and spirituality that leads to ecstasy and deepens intimacy.

I urge you to undertake all of your activities, personal and professional, in the spirit of *seva.* To do so is to live by your heart. Without striving, without effort, you will receive many priceless rewards—including an internal adjustment away from your pain, and perhaps a solution to it altogether. Remember the seventh verse from *The Wisdom of the Tao:* "It is through selfless action that I experience my own fulfillment."

Overcoming Doubt and "God Withdrawal"

One evening, as I was doing my regular meditation, an inspirational wave kept washing over me: "Write about your experience in October 2010 of flirting with atheism and what you learned from it."

For two weeks all I did was read atheist literature of writers like Richard Dawkins and Christopher Hitchens. I read that our existence can be explained by random molecules starting to self-replicate and then evolving, eventually, into humanity. And that we all are in a way atheists as we deny each other's God and religious books, at the same time that many wars have been fought to "prove" whose God is genuine.

Those seemed like good points to me, and at the beginning of the two weeks I felt excited and free. I felt empowered, as though my chains had been cut. But after my initial excitement faded, I started feeling empty, as if something deep inside was missing. I started to have anxiety attacks and felt depressed, lonely, craving God like an addict does when he or she goes into withdrawal. As an ex-pain-management specialist, I know that feeling, and I knew it intimately when I was on pain medication. Hence the title of this section: "God withdrawal." I had stopped meditating, saying mantras, and praying, and in my core I felt hollow. I craved my God fix.

I decided I needed to go deeper. I began to study the ancient wisdom of the East. How could I answer the atheists' reasons for saying God does not exist? I found the answer in nondualistic philosophies which hold that all that exists is consciousness and that all things and beings, including humans, are like waves on an eternal ocean. There is no beginning or end to this pure consciousness. Many universes have come and gone and will come in the future. I learned that there are different levels of consciousness, including individual consciousness, Divine consciousness, and cosmic consciousness. All gods and goddesses are projections of consciousness at the Divine level, like ice formations in ocean water.

Atheists, it would seem, won't believe in any divinity that can't be physically measured by a god-meter. But the very essence of divinity is the fact that it can't be measured. It's beyond the five senses, beyond any physical reference points. It cannot even be adequately described. Further, the theory of the Big Bang is already described in the Buddhist and Hindu traditions of wisdom. Even quantum theory is described in Akashic field concepts. Finally, I believe it is inconceivable that our intelligence and consciousness have arisen from random molecules that somehow started to self-replicate. There has to be an underlying, unifying source.

In the end, the whole experience of "God withdrawal" was very transformative. It deepened my faith in nonreligious spirituality. It connected me to my own deep Inner Truth: We all are the same reality and are connected at a very deep level as waves in the ocean of consciousness. God is not an insurance company from which we can buy protection by praying. We all have been given free will to act as we choose

Now I meditate regularly. I even pray to a "teacher" form of *Shiva,* the Hindu deity who is depicted as an ascetic and mystic but also as a family man with a wife and children. The Hindu deities exist beyond time and the physical world. But now, with my understanding that *Shiva* outside is also *Shiva* inside me, I know that instead of searching for God outside, I need to go deeper inside and learn to listen to the truth and intuition that is there. Even Luke 17:21 in the Bible says, "The Kingdom of God is within you."

With respect to pain, it's impossible to believe that a high degree of spiritual evolution means total freedom from discomfort. Struggle always exists, even if it's struggle to evolve beyond struggle. When the Jewish sage Rabbi Akiva ben Joseph was about to be executed by the Romans in the year 137 BCE, his followers were in despair. Akiva, however, responded that his martyrdom would be the greatest and most satisfying moment of his life. What a sage like Akiva desired was not material comfort or financial success. On the contrary, what causes pain to such people is the absence of opportunity to express their spiritual evolution so they can evolve further.

Fortunately, for those of us who are not at the highest level of spiritual evolution, there are plenty of opportunities for adjustment toward spiritual growth. Taking advantage of those opportunities is the real solution to the challenge of pain.

7

RESOLUTION

In this final chapter of Part Two, we'll look for the last time at the bonds that keep us enslaved to pain and discover how to break them. This will clear the field for Part Three, where we can concentrate on the positive opportunities for freedom at the physical and spiritual levels of our being. In short, by the end of this chapter we will have learned how to clear all forms of negativity, which is essential for resolution. As in Dante's *Divine Comedy,* having passed through the Inferno, we'll be ready to enter a true state of serenity and well-being. But first we must put the barriers behind us. We must recognize the obstacles for exactly what they are and eliminate them from our consciousness and therefore from our lives.

For me, one of the largest obstacles was my assumption concerning pain medications. I assumed that I had no choice but to take, and keep taking, these medication in order to deal with chronic pain. Opiates seemed like the only way. But when I started to meditate, practice yoga, and reduce my stress levels, I found that this assumption was totally wrong. I was able to first reduce my intake of painkillers and gradually come off them entirely.

PAIN CAN BE TRACED TO THREE TYPES OF NEGATIVE THOUGHTS THAT LEAD TO NEGATIVE ACTION

When a patient calls upon a doctor to treat an illness, the doctor is trained to look for certain signs and symptoms that open the way to diagnosis and treatment. In this case the symptoms to look for when treating pain are negative thoughts or emotions that lead to negative action. The Sanskrit word *klesha* perfectly addresses this situation. Its definition is negative thoughts or emotions that are the foundation for negative action. All action originates from thought, although the individual thinker may lose sight of this fact. Many actions are so natural they seem to happen by themselves. We are not, for example, aware of the thought that precedes movement of our hands or feet. But the thought is there, and by slowing down the process of natural physical movement, we can become aware of that thought.

Other, more complex actions originate in thoughts that have become habitual. When these thoughts are severely negative, this can become a painfully self-destructive sequence. Simply, if you expect the worst, the worst will very often happen. Your negative expectation will certainly be an important component of your negative action, and possibly the outright creator of the action. Yet you may have become so habituated to negativity that all this takes place completely outside your conscious awareness. It's like poisoning your body by breathing in a completely colorless, odorless gas that is extremely toxic. Buddhist teachings look at these negative thoughts—these *kleshas*—in a very careful, systematic way. By identifying, clarifying, and categorizing the thoughts, Buddhism brings them into sharp focus so they can be dealt with effectively.

There are many different ways of categorizing the *kleshas* in various Buddhist traditions. One of the most prominent approaches refers to the so-called "Three Poisons" of ignorance, attachment, and aversion. Looking closely at each of the Three Poisons can bring focused consciousness to what has previously been only blind reflex.

Ignorance

In the terminology of the Three Poisons, ignorance refers to a lack of understanding about the basic nature of our life in the world—about what life is and what it isn't. Ignorance is a fundamental wrongheadedness that gives rise to other forms of wrongheaded thinking, including attachment and aversion, the other two poisons.

It's important to understand that ignorance is not at all the same as stupidity. A stupid person lacks the capacity for understanding. Their mental and emotional machine is simply not powerful enough to process the truth. Ignorant people of course have the potential to be enlightened, but what they lack is the necessary information.

This is a problem that can be solved, but it's usually not easy. Even wrong information can seem very convincing. The Greek mathematician and astronomer Ptolemy, who lived in the second century after Christ, created a detailed description of the Earth's place in the center of the universe. Ptolemy's system fully accounted for observable phenomena such as the waxing and waning of the moon and the rising and setting of the sun. Despite this, it was wrong. Yet hundreds of years went by before the error of the Ptolemaic system of cosmology became recognized. Even more remarkable, a significant number of very perceptive individuals actually knew it was wrong, but they had to keep silent or face imprisonment, torture, and death. Some of them did come forward and they paid the price.

In order to achieve a resolution of the pain issues in your life, you need to get beyond the temptations of what has come to be called the Ptolemaic fallacy. You'll have to question the assumptions about yourself and your life that have brought you to this point. And you must aggressively question those assumptions no matter how convincing they seem. Perhaps your assumptions were correct after all, or perhaps not. It's the questioning, not the answers, that make the difference between ignorance and wisdom.

As a way of questioning my assumptions, I evolved an exercise that I can strongly recommend. I call it "One Hundred Questions," and it will require about an hour of your time. Sit quietly and during the next hour write down one hundred questions related to your pain. Just let your thoughts flow, and you'll see that one question leads to another. The key to this exercise is the fact that you don't have to include answers to the questions. That's something you can do at a later time, or maybe not at all. The questions alone—"Why do I have pain?" "Why does my wife not love me?"—will be revealing.

Using this exercise, I was able to see the extreme presence of anger in my life: anger at myself, anger at the world, and even anger at God. I was able to extinguish this anger by my "Triple S Formula," which I also emphatically recommend:

Seva: Service with gratitude.

Sadhana: Daily spiritual practice, including meditation, yoga, or any other spiritually oriented activity you choose.

Sangha: A positive choice to surround yourself with people of high consciousness who can help you advance to that level. To paraphrase Albert Einstein, resolution to a problem cannot be found at the level of consciousness that created the problem.

Attachment

Sometimes when I wake up in the middle of the night, I feel much different than at any time during the day. I have lots of ideas, and I also feel free from distractions. I suspect the reason I have lots of ideas is *because* I'm free from distractions. This insight about distractions has helped me get out of bed at 2:00 A.M. in order to write. It's also helped me, regardless of what time it is. Once you understand the meaning and power of distractions, you can certainly start to live better, too.

What do I mean by a distraction? A distraction is something that diverts your attention, your energy, your mind, your heart, or perhaps your whole being away from the purpose of your life and toward a deceptively attractive alternative. In terms of the *kleshas* and the Three Poisons, a distraction is the enticing energy for connection with the poison of *attachment.*

What exactly makes the alternative *deceptively* attractive? Well, if you could see that alternative's essence, if you could see what it really means and what it can really do to you, you wouldn't find it attractive at all. But since you can't see those inner attributes, you can be distracted and attracted to things that are out of line with your purpose. Not only that, such attachments can be very destructive to your body, your mind, and your spiritual self.

But at first such attachments can be very distracting. At first they can look really good. The concept of "at first" is really important. Attachment in itself is neither good nor bad. If you're attached to learning and growing, to serving and healing, to wisdom and enlightenment, all that is really good. Those attachments never degrade you. They never grow corrupt. They never turn into powerful addictions. The trouble comes when you attach to something with an expiration date—which, unfortunately, does include just about everything that seems really good at first.

I learned that lesson the hard way. Today I'm attached to an intention to share and to serve. As I write that, I'm aware that it may sound pompous or excessively righteous, but there's really no other way to express it. I do want to give value to others from my experiences as a person who has gone through My Dark Night of the Soul. I experienced everything from prostate cancer to chronic pain from a series of surgeries, to dependency on pain medications, to unpredictable, unstoppable, long-term financial loss. But it all looked good at first, so I became distracted and attached to many ticking time bombs, which exploded when their clocks ran down.

Yes, I achieved material wealth, which always includes the possibility of losing it. But it always felt like I never had enough. It was only when I turned my journey inward—when I was *forced* to turn inward—that I found the permanent and imperishable wealth that had been there all along.

Buddhism teaches that attachment to anything that is subject to possible loss can never bring lasting satisfaction. Yes, we are living in the modern world with families, responsibilities, and things that amuse and enliven us. But if we wish to free ourselves from pain, we must learn to engage all that without attachment to it. As the *Bhagavad Gita* teaches, we must learn to firmly establish ourselves in spirit while still taking action in the material world in which we live.

Learning to do this is a really great challenge. One way I'm trying to meet that challenge is by writing this book. Taking positive action while remaining detached from its outcome is essential for bringing resolution to the conflicts and complications that bring pain into our lives. It's a state of being that I call "attached/detached stillness." It's a difficult concept to explain, but I know it when I manage to experience it. With a little practice, I promise you can do that, too.

Aversion

The last of the Three Poisons may be the most interesting. In Sanskrit, it's called *dvesha*, which is usually translated as "aversion" or "repulsion." On the simplest level it's just anger. Whenever we feel rage or aggression toward a person, place, or thing, we've been hooked by an underlying desire for the world to be organized according to our specifications. We just want things to be the way we want them to be.

Your individual personality determines the effect of *dvesha* in your life. Some people go ballistic at the smallest frustration or disappointment. For others, something of greater magnitude is required. A highly evolved soul may be free from aversion altogether, and therefore free from the pain it causes. Strangely, or perhaps not so, the people who have the least to be upset about are often the first ones to get angry. What does that tell us?

On a more philosophical level as well as a more deeply psychological one, the basis of *dvesha* is anger at the phenomenon of change itself. It's not just that something isn't right, but that something might not become right or stay right. Do you have a beautiful house? Did you just buy a nice car? Have you lots of money in the bank? That's wonderful, but are you worried that you paid too much for the house? Or that someone might run into your car? Or that the interest rate on your money might go down? That's aversion, but it's not aversion to the house or the car or the money. It's aversion to what could happen to those possessions in the unpredictable world we live in.

Mingyur Rinpoche, a Tibetan Buddhist spiritual master and prolific author, has written very eloquently about this principle:

> Every strong attachment generates an equally powerful fear that we'll either fail to get what we want or lose whatever we've already gained. This fear, in the language of Buddhism, is known as aversion: a resistance to the inevitable changes that occur as a consequence of the impermanent nature of relative reality.
>
> The notion of a lasting, independently existing self urges us to expend enormous effort in resisting the inevitability of change, making sure that this "self" remains safe and secure. When we've achieved some condition that makes us feel whole and complete, we want everything to stay exactly as it is. The deeper our attachment to whatever this sense of completeness, the greater our fear of losing it.[1]

PART 3

THE ANSWER
TO PAIN

We have explored the process of physical and emotional pain from a practical viewpoint. Crisis, solution, and resolution refer to the dynamics of everyday life. In the book's last three chapters we will discuss responses to pain from a more all-encompassing point of view. Forgiving, loving, and healing transcend the boundaries between the mundane and the spiritual. They even transcend the boundaries that might seem to exist between themselves. Please give close attention to the chapters that follow.

8

FORGIVE

By sharing my thoughts, feelings, and experiences in this book, I want to show how a Dark Night of the Soul can not only pass, but can bring a brighter dawn than ever before. My Dark Night has helped me connect to my inner self, to find the true meaning of my life, and to discover the nature of total wellness. Now I wish to channel all my physical and emotional pain into writings of authentic, timeless value. The dark energies have shifted within me and brought me greater awareness and higher consciousness.

PAST AND FUTURE LIVES

Growing up as a Hindu in India, I was taught to believe in past and future lives. It was just a fact that I had lived before and I would live again. Each incarnation has a purpose, and until that purpose is achieved it must be revisited again and again—after which a new life with a new life's purpose can be addressed.

In the *Bhagavad Gita,* the god and avatar Krishna reveals the true nature of being human. He admonishes the valiant warrior Arjun for hesitating to fight in battle because he is mournful at the thought of taking the lives of other men, even if they are men who have created suffering and pain to the general detriment of the world. Some of these enemies are even Arjun's blood relations.

Krishna is unswerving in the position that there must be a fight to end the prevalence of negative forces. He explains to Arjuna that there is a misapprehension of the human condition—that one can never truly "take" life from another:

> *He who understands him to be the slayer, and he who takes him to be*
> *the slain, both fail to perceive the truth. He neither slays nor is slain.*
> *He says the truth is that within each Human is an eternal Self:*
> *He is never born, nor does he ever die; nor once having been, does*
> *he cease to be.*
> *Unborn, eternal, everlasting, ancient, he is not slain when the body*
> *is slain.*
> —CHAPTER 2, VERSE 19

Krishna explains the cycle of the birth and death of the soul in very simple and straightforward terms:

> *As a man casting off worn-out garments takes other new ones,*
> *So the dweller in the body casting off worn-out bodies takes*
> *others that are new.*
> —CHAPTER 2, VERSE 22

Ultimately we are to understand:

> *Weapons cannot cleave him, nor fire burn him;*
> *Water cannot wet him, nor wind dry him away.*
> —CHAPTER 2, VERSE 23

Celebrated in every aspect of worship and life in India, this understanding of the nature of being human was something I grew up with as a boy. It became a steadfast tenet of my own cultural, social, and philosophical worldview. But as a young man I went to medical school, where I studied the very physically oriented, mechanistic, Western system of health care. I lost all interest in and connection with the concept of the soul and of the possibilities of past lives. These ideas could have no place in the business of wellness or healing; they offered nothing relevant or helpful. As I lost interest, I also discarded the *Gita* scriptures, which in my mind came to represent only ancient superstitions. They could be poetic, they could be beautiful, but they were essentially artifacts from an unenlightened period of history and an uneducated civilization.

Life went on. I came to the United States in 1982 and was still agnostic, or maybe indifferent is a better word. I had no interest in anything of a spiritual nature. Then, as I mentioned in Chapter 1, I injured my right wrist, which led to chronic, unrelenting pain. As a pain management practitioner and a senior anesthesiologist, I of course turned with good and whole faith to various treatments and protocols of Western medicine. I had prescribed these treatments to thousands of patients whom I had cared for over a period of thirty years. These included pain medicines, nerve blocks, and surgery. To my deep distress, none of these treatments worked. Not only did my wrist injury remain unhealed, but the pain remained almost insufferable. There was little or no relief.

This situation involved some comic irony. I was a cardiac anesthesiologist who needed good use of my hands and wrists to administer sensitive doses of pain management medications to people in critical conditions. Now I was off work for almost six months because of chronic pain in my own wrist—and pain management medication was not helping.

My Experience with Past-Life Regression

At that time one of my sisters recommended I read a book titled *Many Lives, Many Masters*. The author of the book, Dr. Brian Weiss, had a very interesting background that in some ways resembled my own. He had an M.D. degree with a specialty in psychiatry. As a mainstream psychotherapist, Dr. Weiss was astonished and skeptical when one of his patients began recalling past-life traumas that seemed to hold the key to her recurring nightmares and anxiety attacks. His skepticism was eroded, however, when she began to channel messages from "the space between lives," which contained remarkable revelations about Dr. Weiss's family and his deceased son. Using past-life therapy, he was able to cure the patient and embark on a new, more meaningful phase of his own career.

I read the book and was fascinated. Professionally, I respected Dr. Weiss as a graduate of Columbia University and Yale Medical School. He was a highly regarded physician like myself. But to be honest, I just couldn't believe what I had read. I decided the book was interesting only as a fairy tale, and I put it aside. Then a coincidence occurred. I went to Phoenix for a conference, and Dr. Weiss also happened to be conducting a workshop there. Out of curiosity, but as a skeptical nonbeliever, I signed up for the workshop. After all, I thought, he has a M.D. degree just as I do, and he's trained at some really impressive schools.

During the workshop, Dr. Weiss took us into a very deep meditation. We were encouraged to travel as far back in time as we needed—even if that meant before our current incarnation. It was a very powerful experience for me. I felt like I was transcending the boundaries of life and death. I seemed to be going back through time.

I remembered two separate lives. In one of them, I was a prince in medieval times. I can still view the setting clearly in my mind. I am standing in the castle courtyard, and there are soldiers with me. I am ordering the soldiers to inflict—and I am personally inflicting—physical punishment on poor peasants in brown tattered clothes. Under Dr. Weiss's direction within that deep meditation, I asked forgiveness from those peasants for what I had done. And they seemed to forgive me.

I found the experience very compelling. Where had all this come from: the vision of myself, the medieval setting, the story, the people, the sense of a very different social system? Had I imagined all this out of nowhere? How? Why? Yes, it had felt very real. But I don't remember it as real, no matter how it felt.

In the second previous life, I was a small boy standing in a crowd and Roman soldiers were dragging Jesus toward the place of his crucifixion. What could that possibly mean? As I got to know Dr. Weiss over time, I once asked about his own past lives. He told me that he too was in that crowd. Since then I have developed a deeper connection with Jesus Christ. I have come to regard Jesus as I also regard Hindu avatars such as Rama and of course our beloved Krishna, who in the *Bhagavad Gita* revealed the essence our human nature.

I am still wondering exactly how all this past-life regression works. I have no explanation for it, given my own Western medical training. But there is no doubt that, strangely enough, something happened shortly after that workshop which astonished my family, my colleagues, and certainly myself. Immediately afterwards, the pain in my wrist began to disappear. Within a few weeks I went back to work. It seemed not just unrealistic, but impossible that I was able to go back in time and ask for forgiveness—and by so doing I could cure the pain in my wrist. Yet that's what seemed to happen.

Past-life regression therapy works just like Freudian analysis or other forms of interpersonal counseling. Patients are regressed back to the point in time where current problems originated. That point is often very far removed from where the patient thinks the issue began, often in a very distant place and in a radically different time. Yet now that far-away cause has surfaced and is having an effect on the patient's life. Once the original starting point has been identified—*in fact, the patient actually re-lives it*—the patient is encouraged to resolve the problem in the setting where it first took place.

Whether we choose to believe in past lives or not, there is now data that, as a therapy, past-life regression works. It is now employed by many psychologists all over the world. Studies are being conducted by researchers at Columbia University and other sites that are seriously exploring the phenomena of past-life recall.

Psychologists who don't care to believe in the concept of past lives can still accept the therapy as useful. Whether the memories are real or imagined, whether they're repressed events or dream-like projections, is not really the point from a therapeutic perspective. What matters is the cathartic release of negative energy in the patient that has lasting positive benefit and often provides relief from a chronic condition in their current life.

The strategy in all forms of regression therapy, past life or not, is that in experiencing painful, hurtful, or difficult memories, we can heal forgotten, disguised, or repressed traumas. Many conventional treatments are useful because at the very least they cause no harm, and they work. In so doing we can release ourselves from the consequences of the injury that is complicating or even running our current everyday experience of the world. In my case, that meant asking forgiveness of the people I had harmed.

I will have more to say about the power of forgiveness, and the power of asking for forgiveness, later in this chapter. But regarding the vision of my medieval incarnation, I have since learned that past-life regression therapy can be a hugely transformational therapeutic treatment. While this emerging field in psychology is open to many questions that have not been definitively answered, I am aware that my experience opened me to the power of therapies for the soul, where in the past I had recognized only therapies for the body. It also revived the belief in spirituality that had been so important to me earlier in life.

To anyone who is in pain, whether it's physical or emotional, the best advice I can give is to keep all options open. If a therapy works, it works. Sometimes, if it's noninvasive and has no negative side effects, we do not have to know exactly how the therapy is working. What's essential is the result. For me, the result was that after going back in time and asking forgiveness, my wrist did heal. After six months of being forced to the sidelines, I was back at work and painfree.

WHAT I'VE LEARNED ABOUT FORGIVENESS AND WHAT I'M STILL LEARNING

Getting through My Dark Night wasn't easy, but I see now there were three emotional and spiritual steps I had to take. The steps sometimes coincided with specific physical actions or events, like asking for forgiveness during past-life regression, but they really existed outside the physical realm. The three steps are quite simply: forgive, love, heal. The steps are separate, but they're part of one spiritual entity. They come together to create a single mantra, one that can be extremely beneficial not only during periods of urgent crisis but also at many other times.

It's easy, and it can even be very tempting, to create a Mini Dark Night of the Soul during every day of your life. It can happen when someone cuts you off in traffic. It can happen to someone else when *you* cut *them* off in traffic. Regardless of the dimensions of the experience, to paraphrase Rudyard Kipling, whether it's a day of doom or a night of drink, the initial feeling is always pretty much the same.

The Role of Blame

The initial feeling is anger, but we need to be more specific than that. It's the special kind of anger called *blame*. You blame God, you blame the Universe, you blame people in your life, and at some deep, often unconscious level you also blame yourself. Anger and blame develop in that exact order, by the way. Blaming goes from the general to the specific, from the macro scale to the micro scale.

From anger and blame directed at God all the way to anger and blame directed at yourself.

It's not easy to forgive a person, and the most difficult person to forgive is *you*. We'll be looking at exactly what forgiveness involves as this chapter goes on. But we can't understand forgiveness without looking at the earlier emotion that makes forgiveness necessary in the first place.

That earlier emotion is blame. There are certainly times when blame is appropriate, especially legal blame. That kind of blaming takes place many times every day. If one person robs another person, the law tries to provide a way to determine who should be blamed. But there are other kinds of blame that exist outside the legal system. And these kinds of blame often cause more pain to the "blamer" than to anyone else.

Very simply, "to blame" means assigning responsibility for some negative outcome. An individual can be legally blamed for causing a car accident. A group of people can be blamed for starting a riot. A tornado can be blamed for destroying a barn. But we don't speak of blaming someone for taking care of a lost kitten or for finding a cure for a disease. The outcome has to be negative in order for blame to come into play.

Blame, like the air, is everywhere. We all do it and sometimes with justification, such as objectively assigning consequences to causes. Your neighbor crashes into your parked car and bears responsibility for the repairs. That's just common sense.

But no matter who may have caused a specific physical event, no matter who is legally responsible, we are always responsible for our own feelings. We must accept that responsibility, or else we are condemning ourselves to playing the role of victim in our own lives. It's your right to blame someone, but you should accept your responsibility for choosing to assign that blame. You can then, perhaps, make a further choice, which would be to forgive the person you blamed. Of course, if you don't make the choice to blame anyone in the first place, then there's no need for forgiveness later on.

Avoiding the impulse to blame demands mental insight and emotional strength. It means going against very powerful and very natural human reflexes. But like so many other important matters, avoiding blame is simple to say but not easy to do. After all, the impulse to blame is very understandable, even justifiable. In everyone's life and throughout human history, there are countless examples of people who deserved blame for their destructive actions, and this includes people who have done a lot more harm than causing a fender bender. There are people for whom merely legal blame doesn't seem to solve the problem.

There are places in the world today in which blame, and revenge, which is the active component of blame, dominate people's lives for generations. Family feuds can continue for a hundred years, long after the original incident is forgotten. This is really a form of mass hypnosis or even mass hysteria. The important point is this: After a certain period of time, what happens to the "bad guys" should not be the primary concern. Focusing on blame, retribution, or even revenge becomes a self-destructive waste of time. We're concerned with the power of forgiveness, which really depends on overcoming the seductive power of blame. Forgiveness becomes possible once you let go of blame. But one form of blame is much more complex than any other and is highly resistant to forgiveness.

Stop Blaming Yourself, Start Forgiving Yourself

We've noted the importance of taking responsibility for your own feelings. While any number of people may be responsible and even blameful for a physical action, what exists in our own minds and hearts are our own credits or our own faults, whatever the case may be. This is especially true as time goes on. If someone causes you serious harm, there is a period of time in which you can credibly say, "That person is making me feel this way." But after many months or many years have gone by, you are the one who is making yourself feel that way. And you need to own up to that.

It may not be easy, but most people are able to connect with these ideas if the concepts of blame and forgiveness are presented correctly. Even people who have been severely victimized during war or criminal activity can come to see the benefits of "letting it go." But blaming yourself is such a potent force, and truly forgiving yourself is so elusive, that a very powerful kind of self-awareness is required. As we continue to examine blame and forgiveness in this chapter, we'll often return to the special category of the internalized form of painful or hurt feelings.

William Faulkner wrote that for everyone born in the South, the date will always be July 3, 1863, and the time will always be ten minutes before 2:00 in the afternoon. That's when the final infantry charge at the Battle of Gettysburg was about to begin. The failure of that charge essentially ended the South's hopes for victory in the Civil War. "The past isn't over," Faulkner wrote in *Requiem for a Nun*. "It's not even past."

That's how it is with many human emotional processes. Time stands still, especially where pain is concerned. Past wounds can infect and even dominate our present and our future. If you were hurt by someone, you may carry blame for many years. You may also blame yourself throughout your lifetime, or you may construct all sorts of protective systems to prevent blaming yourself, and these systems can become so complex that you lose track of where the truth really lies.

We are all in pain. We have all been wounded or damaged in some way, and some of the deepest wounds come from the people closest to us. A wife feels neglected by her husband's concentration on his career. A husband is ashamed when his wife's income is larger than his. A middle-aged woman, the mother of children, is still angry at her own mother for something that happened years ago. A father resents his own father, although that man has been dead for many years. There are an infinite number of variations on this theme, and they all add up to the same thing: anger and blame carried forward indefinitely. The solution and the challenge are to see people— whether they're parents, family members, or the drill sergeant in boot camp —as just that: *people.* Your unconscious mind may see them as monsters, but they are not the ones who pay the price. You pay it.

Anger and blame are static or stagnant conditions. You replay again and again the old hurts and the feelings that were evoked. True forgiveness takes time. It's a cliché to say that something is a journey rather than a destination, but it's true in this case. That can even be a great blessing. Because forgiveness is a process, there's always change. It's a dynamic experience. You can acknowledge that painful things happened to you, or were done to you, but perhaps now you can use that knowledge to make a positive difference in the lives of others and therefore in your own life as well. This doesn't mean you should forget the pain of what was done to you. But if you commit yourself to moving forward, you may be surprised to find that you actually do forget the pain, at least most of the time.

Forgiving can be like mourning. There is pain to begin with, but as the process continues, the pain diminishes. Many people don't realize that the refusal to forgive is an unconscious way of staying in touch with whatever person or thing has caused you pain. You think you want to be rid of them, yet you've found a way to keep thinking about them over and over again.

The mind can be extremely ingenious in making this repetition continue, as in the case of a young woman we'll call Jennifer. Both of Jennifer's parents died while she was young—her mother when she was eight, and her father when she was sixteen. Both of them died of cancer. After her father's death, Jennifer was raised by her stepmother.

Jennifer was a good student, an excellent athlete, and a seemingly well-adjusted young woman through high school and college. But Jennifer always had a secret, something she could tell no one because she knew no one would understand or believe her. Jennifer believed she had cancer. But it was more than that. Jennifer was convinced she had cancer. In her own mind she *knew* she had cancer. But even if she had a full battery of cancer tests and every test was negative, her mind would not be changed. The tests would be wrong. The doctors wouldn't understand. Jennifer had cancer. There was absolutely no doubt in her mind.

What does this story have to do with forgiveness? Jennifer was a classic case of "survivor's guilt." She had seen the parents whom she loved weaken and die—yet she was still alive. She had watched them try to care for her even while their own illnesses worsened. Not only had she survived, but she had matured and grown stronger. So her mind came up with a very creative solution to alleviate the pain in her life. Jennifer convinced herself she had cancer as a form of revenge for her own survival. She blamed herself for outliving her parents, and she could not forgive herself because the whole process was hidden from her. It may seem obvious as we read about it now, but it was completely invisible to Jennifer.

Jennifer could not see how her guilt, and the way her guilt expressed itself through delusions about cancer, was also a way of staying in contact with her parents in an almost physical way. She was sharing a profound physical and emotional experience with them. Although the shared experience was pain and suffering, in an ironic way it kept her parents alive for Jennifer. If she were to forgive herself for survivor's guilt and break away from her cancer hypochondria, there was an unconscious fear that this would represent a final break with her parents. That was something Jennifer was simply not ready to face.

Well into her thirties Jennifer continued to be troubled, and sometimes deeply tormented, by her fear of cancer. Sometimes it would only be in the back of her mind, but there were also days or even weeks when her fear became a constant preoccupation. Then one day, without any apparent warning, Jennifer's dread of cancer approached the dimensions of what is commonly called a nervous breakdown. Alone in her apartment, her hand shook with fear so violently that she was unable to hold a glass of water. Jennifer was sure she was going to die. There was nothing to do but wait for the end. It was too late.

But then something completely unexpected happened. In the same way that this very severe episode of cancer fear started, it stopped. Suddenly Jennifer felt calm, serene, totally at peace. In fact, she was in a very good mood. But that was not all. It wasn't this one episode of hypochondria that ended. Somehow Jennifer realized that her fear was gone forever. Why? She didn't have the answer, just as she had never been able to see why her fear began. It was as if a spell had been broken.

Here's what I think happened. Jennifer was unable to forgive herself, but eventually, after so many years, something deep inside her spirit determined that she had suffered enough. Her last and most painful episode of cancer fear was the final self-punishment her spirit felt she owed herself. Her blame was replaced by forgiveness. Her new life could begin.

THE ART OF FORGIVENESS

The really unfortunate part of Jennifer's story is the amount of suffering she had to endure before she could finally let it go. Perhaps there was no avoiding this. On rare occasions she had confessed her fear to close friends, and even to doctors, all of whom tried to talk her out of it. But she couldn't hear what they were trying to tell her. She wasn't ready.

It doesn't have to be that way. If you're holding onto anger and blame, you must—for your own sake—begin to see what that is costing you. You must also recognize what hidden need you are trying to satisfy. For Jennifer, it was the need to remain connected to her parents and to her survivor's guilt. Ask yourself whether you're caught in that same kind of bind. And be honest with your answers.

Although Jennifer's hypochondria seemed to disappear in a flash, the unconscious process leading up to that moment took more than twenty years to work itself out. Even if you have the power to make a conscious and effective decision toward forgiveness, you may feel that you're not entirely free. That's just the way the human mind and the human heart work in this area. Forgive yourself for that, too!

The process of forgiveness is more of an art than a science. It should be a conscious decision, but there's also an unconscious component that has to come into play. Just like playing a musical instrument or throwing a baseball, it can't be totally analytical. A major league outfielder doesn't calculate the correct angle before he makes a long throw to home plate. Yet a great ballplayer can intuitively hit the target with amazing accuracy. A big part of the reason is simply that he believes he can do it.

Will you forgive yourself? Can you forgive someone whom you don't really *want* to forgive? When you think of something destructive you've done— maybe even something really awful—do you believe other people can genuinely forgive you?

It's really important to do the inner work that will allow you to answer "yes" to those questions. Some people find doing that very difficult. They see their own situations, their own feelings, their own grudges and hurts as just too intense for rational intervention. And they don't see the hidden arrogance that lies behind such things. When a person sees his or her own situation as exceptional, beyond what anyone else has faced, this is basically a form of egotism, even if the situation is extremely painful. Christianity teaches that there are many sins, but the greatest sin is to believe that your guilt is so great that you are beyond God's mercy. But you are not beyond the power of forgiveness. And while there might be two or three people in history who have entered that category, I can confidently say that you aren't one of them.

In my own life, I have had to forgive myself for anything I have done that contributed to My Dark Night. I've had to forgive everyone and everything, including myself, who contributed to my painful circumstances. This fundamentally transformed me. I started to live in the present moment, rather than trapped in past circumstances, or what I wanted them to be in the future. Other people might describe this experience in different terms, but for me it was a matter of forgiving God and all of Creation (including myself) and accepting God's will. I had to surrender to the possibility that the Spirit alone has infinite wisdom.

Finally, here's one dictionary definition of forgiveness:

The process of concluding resentment, indignation, or anger as a result of a perceived offense, indifference, or mistake, or ceasing to demand punishment or restitution.

For help in the very challenging forgiveness process, I have found the famous Serenity Prayer much more useful:

God grant me the serenity
to accept the things I cannot change;
the courage to change the things I can;
and the wisdom to know the difference.

9

LOVE

One day I decided to write about what love means to me. I knew the kind of love I wanted to explore was a feeling that existed between two people, or perhaps more than two. But beyond that I found it difficult to write about love in a conventional essay form. So I tried to imagine some down-to-earth examples:

Love is when a couple can be waiting in line in a store, and just being together is more fun than other people have on their honeymoon.

Love is like what happens when two different flavors of ice cream melt together, and the result is sweeter than either flavor by itself.

Love is when being together is like the fresh smell from the earth as the first rain is falling after a drought.

Love is when, being together, time stops.

Love is when one person happily gives up personal desires in order for another person to be happy.

Love is when people feel that, on this journey called life, they have found their soulmate.

I could compose more maxims like these, but I'm sure you've got the idea. I'm still not able to define love precisely, but there are a few points I can make about it besides the little metaphors you've just read.

I believe, for example, that real love has nothing to do with power, and power resides in the ego in human beings. When people are in love, their egos are at least temporarily on hold. There is no keeping score; there is no envy. Can there be jealousy in the presence of real love? I'm not sure about that, just like I'm uncertain about many things related to love.

Love is fundamentally a state of mind and a feeling in the heart. It in no way depends on any external factors. It is a mental or emotional state of well-being. There may even be moments of euphoria, although those can also be characteristic of infatuation. Any person in the world can be in love, if he or she is truly ready for that experience and meets the right person to share it with.

The source of love is entirely within you. People speak of "finding love," but that doesn't mean you need to look for it. If people in every part of the world and at every station of life can experience real love, we all can. Love is a potential ability that exists within every individual. You can be in love despite any obstacles, or perhaps because of them, as in *Romeo and Juliet*. Like the principles of quantum mechanics, there is no denying that love exists, yet it's also a complete mystery. As Emily Dickinson wrote, "It's all we know of heaven." And she added, "And it's all we need of hell." Maybe she was just having a bad day.

ABOVE ALL, LOVE MAKES PEOPLE HAPPY

Just as love is an elusive concept to define, the happiness that love creates is also mysterious. But as with love, some observations can be made. Positive emotions and thoughts make us happy. Optimism invites love. A person in love experiences life in a positive way and needs no further reason to be happy. An incident of sadness will not make that person sad for very long, because sadness cannot persist for long in the presence of love. Happiness and love

100

work in tandem. Love doesn't mean that you become completely disengaged from the realities of life, or from any desire to change your situation in life for the better. But in a fundamental way you are happy with what you have. Being content puts your worries to rest and gives you reason to be happy.

Love begets happiness, so pain cannot coexist with it. But again we need to distinguish happiness from euphoria. Love is very grounded, while euphoria is a high. Happiness depends on your attitude. Even if you have all the money in the world, but if you deal with people and situations with a negative mindset, you'll not be happy within. Blindly trying to achieve irrational wishes or fulfill unreasonable desires repels both happiness and love. Reaching for the sky is good, but being honest with ourselves is better.

Love inspires accomplishment, and accomplishment fosters happiness. Happiness is the reward for achieving your aims, targets, and goals. It's a form of appreciation for your successful values and beliefs. It helps to have plenty of short-term goals, so you've many accomplishments in life. That will help cultivate long-term happiness.

Love creates openness and acceptance, and acceptance allows happiness. Whatever has happened cannot be undone. A bell can't be unrung. Accept whatever happened because it had to happen, and accept that there is a reason behind everything that occurs. This acceptance represents a decision to relinquish power. Just as love cancels out any power struggle with another person, acceptance blocks power struggles with the Universe itself.

Love nurtures forgiveness, and forgiveness nurtures happiness. We've discussed the importance of forgiveness as a way to grow and move forward by clearing our heart and mind of negative feelings. We need to keep smiling as that keeps the body in a condition of minimum stress and creates reasons for happiness to dwell within. A happy person is most likely to be healthy, free of stress and all kinds of cardiovascular and other degenerative problems.

Love gives rise to a sense of purpose, and purpose promotes happiness. A sense of purpose instills a feeling of usefulness and satisfaction. Everybody has a spiritual purpose, and you need to know yours. Indulge in trying to know yourself better, define your life's purpose, and work toward it. That will make you happy.

Love for family and friends creates happiness in life, so stay close to and nurture the people who are important in your life. Happy people are found to have more rewarding social ties than unhappy ones. Sharing happiness makes us feel better, and marriage is one relationship where sharing, caring, and love lay the foundation for a happy life. However, even if a relationship goes sour, you need to move on and be optimistic about what's in store for you in the future.

Love makes a good life possible, and a good life attracts happiness. This does not necessarily mean having money or status. It's about how you live your life, your thoughts and deeds. Being kind, generous, helpful, and good to others creates long-lasting, happy memories, especially when nothing is expected in return. After all, happiness is not something that is experienced like pleasure; it is carried in our memories and may be remembered forever. Having an attitude of gratitude toward all and living in the present allow us to cherish all positive relationships, pleasures, and moments in life.

A study by the Harvard Business School postulates that being able to spend money on others makes people happier than spending it on themselves. According to the Greek philosopher Aristotle, happiness is "the practice of virtue with reason."

Another apt quote is from Abraham Lincoln: "Most people are about as happy as they make up their mind to be." The subtlest component of happiness seems to be thought; just as the essence of love is feeling. We become what we think, and we also become what we feel. Right thinking and right feeling are the best seeds for planting, so there can be a harvest of love and happiness in life that will remain forever.

10

HEAL

I want to tell you a story that could well be my life story, but it isn't. Vijay is a first-generation immigrant from India. After receiving a degree in mechanical engineering, he came to the promised land of America in 1982. Vijay worked hard to achieve the so-called American Dream: a big house, an expensive car, a huge-screen television, and all the rest. Yet the urge to get ahead kept driving him harder and harder. Until recently, he typically worked sixty or more hours a week, often bringing paperwork home to try to catch up on weekends, which meant minimal family time.

After thirty-one years of working the American Dream, Vijay had begun to realize that he was short-changing both his family's life and his own by always stretching himself to move higher and higher up the rungs of the corporate ladder. But now the fact that he had been ignoring his family became clearer to him than ever before: It really hit home.

As a result, stress had become a major player in his life. His wife, Lina, expressed her concerns about this many times, but Vijay ignored her. Now the stress, compounded by lack of exercise, unhealthy eating habits, and poor sleep, was taking a severe physical toll. When he had been in college, Vijay had weighed a trim 155 pounds. Now he was above 200. Worse, he had developed high blood pressure and diabetes mellitus. Eventually, he decided he needed a break so he traveled to South Asia with his family.

One day Vijay was walking alone. As he strolled past a muddy swamp, he saw a beautiful lotus flower in the middle of the water. He knew about the lotus flower, which grows across South Asia and is often referred to in Asian literature. He stopped and gazed at the beautiful red and pink lotus for a few minutes, thinking about how peaceful it seemed out there in the murky water. Then he had an epiphany. "Live in the world like a lotus," he said aloud. "This is what I should do. Life is full of murky waters—worries, problems, circumstances that must be dealt with. What I need to do is learn how not to become immersed in those waters. I must learn how to be above them, how to float on them, like the lotus."

As he meditated on this experience, Vijay realized the value of having one's so-called "thermostat of happiness" set high. His expectation of life should be joyful, difficult though that might sometimes seem, and with time that expectation would have a positive influence on reality. By creating positive expectations, Vijay was able to float above the difficult challenges that life presented him. His life became more joyful; he experienced daily bliss. He became more productive, more creative, more of a team player. He was surprised that he got promoted to be senior vice president, the position he had sought when trying to work harder and harder. His personal health and his family life also improved tremendously. He was free from pain. He was well. He was healed.

WHAT HEALING MEANS

Healing is a term we hear a lot these days. People use the word when referring to both physical and emotional processes. We know that healing denotes something very desirable, something we should all be seeking. But what, really, is healing? Many people mistake healing as simply the removal of disease. But real healing goes much deeper.

Some might say that healing refers to physical health and leave it at that. But many people who are physically healthy are also stressed, lonely, fearful, and unhappy. Clearly, these people are far from healed. That's because healing includes much more than just physical health.

I've written a book entitled *The Soul of Wellness*. But as much as I'm interested in and respectful of the condition of being well, healing is actually a much more dynamic process. It's also much more challenging. A person can be well without ever being ill, but in order to heal, people have to undergo a physical or emotional test. They have to be sick in order to get well, and the passage between those two conditions is healing.

Let me make a very personal distinction between two words that many people use interchangeably: curing and healing. When we speak of someone being cured, that means the presence of disease has been removed. The individual is returned to the condition he or she was in before the onset of the illness. But returning someone to their prior condition does not, in my opinion, constitute healing. A healed person is one who is fundamentally different than he or she was in the past. A healed person is always in flux, always changing, because healing is a process, while being cured is a static condition.

Healing, because it is ongoing, requires continuing attention and effort. It's transformation. One could even say it's a miracle. In the New Testament, Jesus does not busy himself with helping well people continue their state of wellness. Instead, he heals the sick, and those who watch this consider it miraculous. What's more, Jesus makes it clear that the healing process is an internal process on the part of those who need to be healed. Jesus creates the setting in which the healing will take place, but when it happens, he doesn't take credit for it.

Though some might not admit it, every doctor knows that this is exactly what modern medicine does as well. We create the physical setting in which the body's natural healing powers are able to operate. There are some diseases that we are actually able to cure, but for the most part our job is removing obstacles to healing.

That's also what I've attempted to do with this book. I have no illusions that words on a page, in and of themselves, can bring an end to pain or to any other biomechanical problem. But it is possible, in my opinion, for words to lead you to take action on your own behalf—to make positive changes in how you live your life and to replace self-destructive habits with positive ones. At the very least, I urge you to question why you need self-created obstacles that stand between who you are now and who you could be when you are healed.

I will never know whether the book has succeeded in achieving its purpose. But just knowing that this was my intention is a healing experience for me. If the book also inspires you to begin healing, that is truly a blessing for both of us.

ENDNOTES

Chapter 1. "I Feel Your Pain"

1. International Association for the Study of Pain. www.iasp-pain.org.

2. "The Mirror-Neuron Study," 2004. psych.colorado.edu/~kimlab/Rizzolatti.annurev.neuro.2004.pdf.

Chapter 2. Life as Pain or Life as Love?

1. Anapol, Deborah. *The Seven Natural Laws of Love.* Fulton, CA: Elite Books, 2005.

2. MacCoby, Nathan, and Farquhar, John W. "Communication for Health: Unselling Heart Disease." *Journal of Communication* Vol. 25/3 (September 1975): 114–126.

3. U.S. Department of Health and Human Services. "The Effects of Marriage on Health." June 2007. http://aspe.hhs.gov/hsp/07/marriageonhealth.

4. Fisher, Dr. Helen. www.helenfisher.com.

Chapter 3. Masking Pain

1. ABC News. "Prescription Painkiller Use at Record High for Americans." April 20, 2011. abcnews.go.com/US/prescription-painkillers-

record-number-americans-pain-medication/story?id=13421828#.UX
gtiLUU8_Y.

2. Centers for Disease Control. "Prescription Painkiller Overdoses in the U.S." November 2011. http://www.cdc.gov/vitalsigns/Painkiller Overdoses/.

Chapter 6. Adjustment

1. Dyer, Wayne W. *Getting to the Gap.* Carlsbad, Calif.: Hay House, 2002.

2. Frederickson, Dr. Barbara. www.unc.edu/peplab/barb_frederickson_page/html.

Chapter 7. Resolution

1. Rinpoche, Mingyur. *The Joy of Living: Unlocking the Secret and Science of Happiness.* New York: Three Rivers Press, 2008.

FURTHER READING

Many current books deal with drugs and surgery as options for controlling chronic pain. The list below is intended to provide spiritual as well as practical advice, with emphasis on Ayurvedic and Buddhist teachings.

Alter, Robert. *The Wisdom Books: Job, Proverbs, and Ecclesiastes: A Translation with Commentary.* New York: W.W. Norton, 2011.
A clear and accurate translation of three books of the Bible by a leading scholar.

The Bhagavad Gita, trans. Eknath Easwaran. Tomales, CA: Nilgiri Press, 2nd ed., 2007.
A very accessible translation of the most fundamental book of Indian spirituality.

Chopra, Deepak. *Perfect Health: The Complete Mind/Body Guide.* New York: Harmony Books, 2001.
The best introduction to Ayurvedic principles and practices.

The Dalai Lama. *The Art of Happiness, 10th Anniversary Edition: A Handbook for Living.* New York: Riverhead Books, 2009.
The art of replacing pain with joy through spiritual wisdom.

_____. *Stages of Meditation*. Boston: Snow Lion Books, 2003.
The best overview of the meditation experience.

Egoscue, Pete. *Pain Free: A Revolutionary Method for Stopping Chronic Pain*. New York: Bantam Books, 2000.
A Western approach to chronic pain control without drugs or surgery.

Frawley, Dr. David. *Ayurvedic Healing: A Comprehensive Guide*. Twin Lakes, WI: Lotus Press, 2001.
An extremely detailed guide by a thoroughly knowledgeable authority.

_____. *The Yoga of Herbs: An Ayurvedic Guide to Herbal Medicine*. Twin Lakes, WI: Lotus Press, 1986.
A concise encyclopedia of herbs and their applications for specific health issues.

_____, and Summerfield Kozak, Sandra. *Yoga for Your Type: An Ayurvedic Approach to Your Asana Practice*. Twin Lakes, WI: Lotus Press, 2001.
Yoga from the perspective of Ayurvedic body types.

Lad, Vasant. *Ayurveda: The Science of Self Healing: A Practical Guide*. Twin Lakes, WI: Lotus Press, 1993.
A philosophical and practical guide to Ayurvedic self-care.

Langer, Ellen. *Mindfulness*. Cambridge, MA: Da Capo Press, 1990.
A Harvard professor's breakthrough study of mindful awareness.

Simon, David, M.D. *The Wisdom of Healing: A Natural Mind Body Program for Optimal Wellness*. New York: Three Rivers Press, 1998.
A neurologist's integration of Ayurvedic and Western approaches to healing.

Tsering, Geshe Tashi. *The Four Noble Truths: The Foundation of Buddhist Thought*, vol. 1. Somerville, MA: Wisdom Publications, 2005.
An explanation of the most fundamental Buddhist teachings.

Yogananda, P. *Autobiography of a Yogi*. London: Rider Books, 1955.
One of the most influential and most widely read books on spirituality.

ONLINE RESOURCES

Internet websites are always in flux, but these are most likely to be permanent and readily accessible.

The AARP website has an article on chronic pain by Dr. Mehmet Oz.
www.aarp.org/health/conditions-treatments/info-07-2012/treating-chronic-pain-without-drugs-oz.html

The American Chronic Pain Association, "the voice of people with pain."
www.theacpa.org

The State of California's complete but somewhat technical inventory of chronic pain treatments.
www.dir.ca.gov/dwc/DWCPropRegs/MTUS_Regulations/MTUS_ChronicPainMedicalTreatmentGuidelines.pdf

The Centers for Disease Control offers a section on pain medication facts.
www.cdc.gov/Features/VitalSigns/PainkillerOverdoses

Deepak Chopra's website has several sections on treating chronic pain.
www.chopra.com

The International Association for the Study of Pain.
www.iasp-pain.org//AM/Template.cfm?Section=Home

The Internet Drug List offers a comprehensive discussion of pain medications.
www.rxlist.com/script/main/art.asp?articlekey=104699

The National Institutes of Health offers information on chronic pain.
www.ninds.nih.gov/disorders/chronic_pain/chronic_pain.htm

Psychology Today *provides an overview of chronic pain.*
www.psychologytoday.com/basics/chronic-pain

An outstanding yoga instructor with expertise in yoga for chronic pain.
www.yogicameron.com/

INDEX

Roosevelt, Franklin D., 28
Rumi (poet), 55

S

Sadhana, 76
Samskara, 46
Sangha, 76
Sattva, 42
Self, 54, 79
 awareness of, 22–23, 92
 connection to, 23–24
 Higher, 21–24, 25, 55, 56
 See also Soul.
Separateness, 53
Serenity Prayer, 97
Service, selfless. See *Seva.*
Seva, 48, 68, 76
Sex, 69
Shiva (god), 71
Shock, 57, 58
Smiling, 101
Soul, 15, 17, 42, 55, 56, 84, 88
 software for, 45–48
 See also Self, Higher.
Soul of Wellness, The (Parti), 105
Spending, 102
Spiritual enlightenment, 15,
 21–22, 54, 63–64, 67, 70–72,
 76, 78
Spiritual practice, 76
Spirituality, 71, 78, 88, 96–97,
 102
Stimuli, 8
Stress, 19, 43, 66, 101

Success, 22–24
 material, 22, 62–63, 78, 79
Support, emotional, 19–20, 102
Sympathy, 12

T

Tamas, 42
Thankfulness, 59
Therapies, 88–89
Thoughts, 39, 61, 93–94, 102
 negative, 74
Three Poisons, 74–79
Tolle, Eckhart, 55
Touch, human, 19
Toxins, 17, 34, 43, 44, 45
Triple S Formula, 76

V

Vasansa, 46
Vasopressin, 19
Vata dosha, 44
Vicodin, 30
Victims, 90, 92

W

Weber, Max, 63
Weiss, Brian, 8586, 87
Wellness, 105
Wisdom of the Tao, The, 70
Withdrawal, 57

Y

Yama (god), 55–55
Yoga, 21, 25, 35–36, 44, 67, 76

ABOUT THE AUTHOR

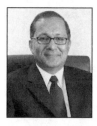 **Rajiv Parti, M.D.**, is a specialist in pain management with more than thirty years clinical experience. He was chief of anesthesiology at Bakersfield Heart Hospital where he specialized in cardiac anesthesia for fifteen years. Dr. Parti founded the Pain Management Institute of California in Bakersfield in 2007, and under his direction it has served thousands of patients for relief of acute and chronic pain.

Dr. Parti's personal experience with life-threatening health challenges led him to explore the healing potential of complementary and alternative medicine. His study and practice of Ayurveda, yoga, meditation, and other Eastern traditions have earned him the same rigorous expertise that he achieved as an allopathic doctor. Dr. Parti recently stepped down from full-time clinical practice to concentrate on his own recovery and to write. He is working with his colleagues at the Pain Management Institute of California on the benefits of meditation and yoga for pain management.

Dr. Parti's first book, *The Soul of Wellness,* is available at amazon.com.